Coping with and Surviving
Mouth, Head and Neck Cancers

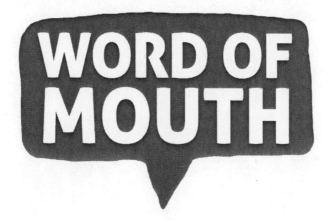

Dedication

DEDICATED TO ALL THOSE WHO are currently fighting cancer: the people who are directly affected, their families and supporters, and the medical teams who treat and care for them.

Coping with and Surviving
Mouth, Head and Neck Cancers

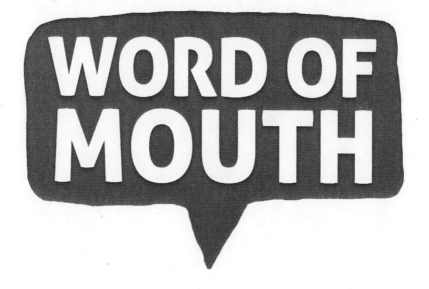

WORD OF
MOUTH

Edited by

Denise MacCarthy and Lia Mills

First published in 2013 by Word of Mouth Publishing
E-mail: wordofmouthimprint@gmail.com
Text © 2013 individual contributors
Internal illustrations © Irish Cancer Society and Shutterstock

Paperback   ISBN: 978-1-909483-31-6
Ebook – Mobi format   ISBN: 978-1-909483-32-3
Ebook – ePub format   ISBN: 978-1-909483-33-0

A CIP catalogue record for this book is available from the British Library.

Produced by Kazoo Independent Publishing Services
222 Beech Park, Lucan, Co. Dublin
www.kazoopublishing.com

Kazoo Independent Publishing Services is not the publisher of this work. All rights and responsibilities pertaining to this work remain with Word of Mouth Publishing.

Index by Dr Laurence Errington
Cover design by Andrew Brown
Cover illustration: www.shutterstock.com
Printed in the EU

Contents

PART THREE

Food, Eating and Recipes

PART FOUR

Foreword

MOUTH, HEAD AND NECK CANCERS are very important diseases. The prognosis for these cancers when they present early is very good, but unfortunately, despite awareness programmes, they often present late, with a much poorer prognosis. This book explains, in an easily readable and patient-friendly manner, the role of all the supporting team members who will be involved in the provision of care. It is an important step forward in the war against this cancer and it is an essential read for anyone who has been diagnosed with mouth, head and neck cancer.

Throughout their treatment patients get to know the surgeons (ear nose and throat, maxillofacial, and plastic surgeons), the radiation oncologists, the medical oncologists, and the other supporting team members (allied health professionals). They are often surprised at the extent and importance of the part played by each team member of the multidisciplinary team (MDT). The number of people a patient needs to see can be frightening – too much information in a very short time can be overwhelming. This book will help to deal with that overload. Treatment of mouth, head and neck cancers does not work unless the whole team and the community work together with the same goal of providing the best possible patient care. There is no room for egos, and all team members are encouraged to express their views. All proper investigations are completed, and after every member of the MDT meets, a proposed treatment plan is agreed. The patient is informed of the discussion and the treatment that is recommended. The patient must ultimately decide. The MDT sets standards, allows peer review, and breaks down barriers between different groups. It also allows international comparisons to be made and provides a forum for discussion of the best treatments currently available. The stories of patients in this book highlight that the MDTs have been successful. If the patient is not happy with the discussions and treatment recommended, a second opinion is sought. Teams need to be treating enough mouth, head and neck cancer patients to allow proper assessment of treatment outcomes.

If the potential army of the general public, doctors, dentists, pharmacists and allied health professionals can be made more aware of the signs and symptoms of mouth, head and neck cancer, there is a chance of improving the outcome through early diagnosis. This could save patients a huge amount of advanced cancer treatment and be very cost-effective for the HSE. As highlighted by the personal stories from patients, too often we see new patients who have been sent back and forth between two or three doctors or dentists. This delays the eventual diagnosis, and subsequent investigations and treatments. A mouth, head and neck examination takes less than five minutes. Education is essential for prevention.[1]

Head and neck cancer affects 300–400 people each year in Ireland. (This number does not include thyroid cancer.) It affects all levels of society but more often the less well off, which can create sometimes seemingly insurmountable problems for patients. It usually affects people over fifty and is more common in men but, as you can see in the very well-written patient stories, it can affect any age or gender. There is often a smoking and alcohol history but again this is not always the case, and patients are devastated when, despite having stopped smoking or never having smoked, they develop the disease. It is not a well-publicised cancer like breast, lung or prostate cancer and therefore despite the great efforts of patients, the staff of the two Dental Hospitals, the Irish Dental Association, the Irish Cancer Society and the Dental Health Foundation, it has not been prioritised by the HSE. It has to a large extent been the 'Cinderella cancer' in the HSE, with little funding for the support services required for these disadvantaged patients. Oral and dental rehabilitation with dental implants, particularly for those patients requiring radiotherapy, chemotherapy or extensive jaw resections, should be available through HSE earmarked funding or medical cards, and it is not.

The diagnosis, investigation and management of mouth, head and neck cancer are very challenging for the whole team. The support of family, friends and the clinical staff is essential during this time. Surgery is the mainstay of treatment for mouth cancer and radiotherapy is the mainstay of treatment for throat (laryngeal) cancer. The consequences of mouth, head and neck cancer treatment are highlighted by the different allied health professional specialties contributing to our patients' care. Any cancer is distressing for a patient, however a cancer that might cause any or all of the following is a huge stress for patients: facial disfigurement, loss of smell, taste, speech, vision or hearing, dry mouth, loss of ability to talk, limited jaw or neck movement, loss of teeth and ability to eat, loss of swallowing and loss of sensation to the face or neck.

Every patient is different and every treatment will have to be individually planned to treat their cancer; this is done at the MDT meetings. Each type or combination of treatment (surgery, radiotherapy and chemotherapy) also has different immediate and long-term consequences. Fortunately, our patient stories highlight that each person's experience is unique, and that even though some of

---

1. MacCarthy, D. (2011) Oral and neck examination for early detection of oral cancer – a practical guide. *Journal of the Irish Dental Association.* 57 (4). p.195–199.

these consequences occur, the patient usually improves with time by learning to cope or by following the constructive advice given in this book. It is important to seek help early and not to be afraid to ask difficult questions. The patient stories highlight the need for clinical honesty, trust between the patient and the clinical team, and empathy rather than sympathy. The aim is to provide the highest standard of treatment available for oral rehabilitation (speech, normal eating and swallowing), and to decrease or eliminate the consequences of some of the treatments.

Sometimes all we can offer is palliation, but even when this is the case we need to do it well so that patients know and feel that they will be treated with dignity and respect. There is also a need for improved support for bereaved families and carers, if it should happen that a person dies.

This book is all about the patients, highlighting the extended team of people available to them, giving them tips from patients' personal experiences – what worked for them – and most importantly giving advice on how to work with the system to ensure they receive the best care possible. Thanks on behalf of future mouth, head and neck cancer patients to all those who contributed to this book. Thanks also to the Molar Rollers who helped fund this project so that *Word of Mouth* can be available to all mouth, head and neck cancer patients.

It has been a very rewarding experience working with the team highlighted in this book and in particular with the patients. Seeing them come back to the clinic, beat the odds, eating, drinking and speaking, makes it all worth while.

There is still a lot of work to do and this book is one big step in the right direction.

Prof Leo F. A. Stassen
National Maxillofacial Unit, St James's Hospital, Dublin
August 2013

Acknowledgements

THE INSPIRATION AND MOTIVATING FORCE behind this book has been the very many strong, courageous people we've encountered over the years in the strange and often surreal world of mouth, head and neck cancer; our first thanks go to them.

That world would be a bleaker, scarier place without the small army of medical and dental professionals who are brave and dedicated enough to stand beside those who are ill and help them to face the demands of treatment. We'd especially like to acknowledge the work of Professor Donal Hollywood, who treated many of the contributors and was a colleague to others, and whose recent death is such an enormous loss to all of us.

In particular, we want to thank all the people who supported Word of Mouth by giving freely of their time, insight and expertise. We would especially like to thank our contributors. Some of them preferred not to be identified, but they know who they are. If we have forgotten anyone, we apologise.

Thanks to Ann Allen, Nick Austin, Valerie Bailey, Barbara Bolton, Donna Bond, Tony Carlin, Allison Connolly, Agnella Craig, Martina Delaney, Charles Dobbyn, Joanne Dowds, Bernie Dwyer, Joseph Furlong, Patricia Gannon, Aoife Gorham, Therese Harvey, Sandra Keating, Michael Keenan, Rory Kelly, Jacinta Kendrick, Adrian Kennedy, Rita Kierce, Anne L'Hénoret, James Lucey, Anne McCaffrey, Lionel McCarthy, Margaret McGrath, Philip McKeon, Reginald MacMahon, Jean-Marc Monseux, Edward Morrall, William Murray, Edward Naessens, Joy Norton, Hannah O'Driscoll, Suzanne O'Leary, Noreen O'Regan, Gayle Pierce, Ian Quigley, Noel Reilly, Stefan Sipka, Natalia Sipkova, Wenda Thomas, Sarah Troute, Melina Venkova, Róisín Whelan, Ben Wu. We'd also like to thank their families and friends, especially because we had to leave out many individual expressions of thanks – not only to families, but to individual dentists, doctors and nurses as well – for logistical reasons.

The families of the editorial group, too, have been incredibly patient while the work has been in progress. They've had a lot to put up with. You're brilliant, and we couldn't have done it without you.

Other supporters are too numerous to mention individually but we'd like to acknowledge in particular the continuing and generous support of Professors Leo Stassen, June Nunn and Stephen Flint, Doctors Osama Omer, Mary Clarke, Mary Collins, Veronica Fisher and Mr Kumara Ekanayake at the Dublin Dental University Hospital. We'd also like to acknowledge the dedication and hard work of Mouth, Head and Neck Cancer Awareness Ireland (MHNCAI) who initiated a national awareness campaign in 2010 and continue to run it (go to www.mouthcancerawareness.ie for details of the latest campaign). The group comprises individuals who have come through mouth, head and neck cancer treatment and staff from the Dublin Dental University Hospital, Cork University Dental Hospital, the Dental Health Foundation, and the Irish Dental Association, working with the support of the Irish Cancer Society.

We got strong guidance from everyone at Kazoo Independent Publishing Services, with special thanks to Robert Doran for the patient copy-editing. Thanks also to Professor Derry Shanley and Dr Brendan Glass for reading and commenting on the manuscript.

Without the generous support of John Hammond and the Molar Rollers the book would not have been possible.

The editorial group who gave their time voluntarily to help with the book are: Bernie Dwyer, Denise MacCarthy, Lia Mills, Edward Naessens, Dalva O'Brien, Wenda Thomas, Sarah Troute and Róisín Whelan. We have been saddened by the loss of Bernie Dwyer, who died while we were in the process of editing. She brought her own particular vivacity and enthusiasm to the project. We miss her.

Denise MacCarthy and Lia Mills

The Molar Rollers

THE MOLAR ROLLERS CYCLING GROUP was founded late in 2009 by cycling devotees from among the staff and friends of the Dublin Dental University Hospital. Cyclists of all abilities were encouraged to join the weekend spins from the Phoenix Park.

A year later a fund-raising cycle to London was decided upon. In August 2011, 31 riders and support crew were given an enthusiastic send-off from DDUH, and eight days and 600 km later the safe arrival of all was celebrated at St Thomas' Hospital at Westminster Bridge.

Through individual and corporate sponsorship, €60,000 was raised and distributed by the Molar Rollers board of trustees. Many individual cancer patients benefited from funds allocated to them through GPs and other healthcare specialists.

The residual funds were then set aside to help defray the costs of this admirable and unprecedented publication.

The Molar Rollers are immensely proud to be associated with this project and we congratulate the editorial group on its accomplishment.

John Hammond and Professor Brian O'Connell

Introduction

IF YOU ARE READING THIS, the chances are that you, or someone you care about, have been diagnosed with some form of mouth, head and neck cancer. Every year between 300 and 400 people are diagnosed with these diseases in Ireland. The incidence is growing, especially among younger people; yet many only hear about these diseases for the first time when they get their own diagnosis. If you are one of these people, you are probably feeling a complicated range of emotions, from shock through confusion and worry to downright fear.

You want to know what will happen. You've had your first in a long series of meetings with a bewildering number of medical personnel, many completely new to you. It has probably dawned on you that the treatment of mouth, head and neck cancer is a complicated business. That's why we felt that a general guide, written by people who have been treated for the disease and by the professionals involved in their care, would be helpful.

The first thing we want to stress is that no two cancers are the same and no two people have the same experience of cancer. This is especially true of mouth, head and neck cancers because of the number of different sites where cancer may be found, the structure and function of those sites, the different types of cancer and the different stages at which diagnosis takes place.

While we're on the subject of individual experience, we'd like to point out that if you go on the internet to research your new diagnosis, you may find yourself overwhelmed by statistics. Please remember that you don't have all the information you need to interpret those figures, and even more importantly, that those figures know nothing whatsoever about you. Numbers have a way of looking as if they know what they're talking about, but in fact they don't know anything about your genetic make-up, your personal circumstances, diet or general health. They don't know a thing about luck. So look at them if you must, and then forget them.

Because the disease is relatively unknown, many people are diagnosed late, which complicates matters. Some people sail through treatment and barely register that they have the disease at all. For others it's not so easy.

Who are we?

We are a group of patients and staff of the Dublin Dental University Hospital who came together to compile a book that would be helpful to mouth, head and neck cancer patients. The book has been generously funded by the Molar Rollers, a group of Dental Hospital staff who raised funds in 2011 by cycling from Dublin to London. They were motivated to raise the money following the first Mouth, Head and Neck Cancer Awareness Day held in Ireland, in 2010. We can't thank them enough.

We approached a small number of patients and asked them to write the story of their cancer. Then we asked people who work in the field to offer their perspective on what a person might encounter along the way. Again, we want to stress that just because one or two people in this book experienced *X* or *Y* does *not* mean that you will.

One of the first things people discover after their diagnosis is that there is a new, highly specialised language to learn. People, specialities, tests and procedures come attached to words you've never heard before. A large team of dedicated people is involved from referral, through assessment, diagnosis, treatment, rehabilitation and long-term post-treatment support. It can be hard to keep track of who's who and what their role is. A common piece of advice in the memoirs is to bring another person and/or a notebook with you to appointments. Ask the team to explain the things you don't understand. Ask them to spell the words. Write down what they tell you. There will be so much going on in your head that you will forget or confuse things if you don't.

It wasn't possible to cover every aspect of treatment. Given the disparity between cases, it would be difficult for a surgeon or an oncologist, for example, to give an account of routine treatment, because the disease is not routine and specialists prefer to give specific explanations tailored to specific people and treatment plans.

In the memoirs, we avoided naming individual practitioners, but we couldn't avoid naming the hospitals. Many contributors made detailed statements of thanks and appreciation to particular individuals, but we didn't include these, other than in a general way. Nearly everyone said how much they appreciated their families and friends who supported them through treatment, and acknowledged the importance of that support. Many individuals were named; again, space dictated that we couldn't include these. But here are two examples:

'When it was all over I remember thinking that I had not realised how much I was loved by my family and friends. They were suffering as well but kept it very much between themselves so as not to upset me. Those of us with families are certainly blessed because of all the love and support they bring us at a time like this.'

Bernie Dwyer

'My brother was fortunate that he had a supportive family and wonderful friends who helped him through his illness. I took on the role of carer when it came to medication, hospital appointments and helping him build up his strength again. He was self-employed and lost his business as a result of the illness, so there was a lot of form-filling and telephone calls to ensure some financial aid, which he was too ill to organise himself. My concern would be that patients without family support would fall through the net, so I really hope the HSE have some kind of system in place to prevent this happening.'

Valerie Bailey

Beyond these omissions, we have tried not to interfere with the individual character of the stories people wrote. This means that the tone and style varies throughout the book. Some are darker than others, while some are almost giddy. We felt that this is an accurate reflection of the different experiences people have on this journey. It was not our job (or our intention) to censor anyone; it would have been counter-productive to try.

Many people had positive experiences along the way. Others describe the pressure they felt to look for the positive and to 'be strong'. The reality for most is more complex, as expressed here:

'I'd love if we could highlight a concept that is evident in pretty much all of the submissions but tends to get overlooked when it comes to a cancer experience. The public discourse tends to be too much focus on fear, tragedy, trauma, and crisis. Whereas many survivors experience something called post-traumatic growth.

'I'd prefer every time, were I given the choice, not to have had cancer. But the truth is that it also helped me grow stronger, having pulled through the worst of it. In terms of talking to a person who is going through treatment I feel it is important to let them know that there is light at the end of the tunnel. There is a future, and there can be surprising and good realisations and breakthroughs along the way.'

Edward Naessens

How were the contributors chosen?

People who were more than one year post-treatment were asked if they would be interested in contributing a memoir. The request was made informally when individuals attended for routine follow-up at the Dublin Dental University Hospital in early 2013. There was an 80 per cent positive response.

Thirty-four people contributed their own stories, 18 women and 16 men. Thirty-two were cancer survivors and two were family members or carers. The age range was 19 to 73. The time period which had elapsed since cancer diagnosis ranged from two years to 21 years. Eighteen of the group came from Dublin, 12 from Leinster, three from Munster and one from Connaught. There were four contributors who had moved to Ireland in recent years.

The types of mouth, head and neck cancer were: squamous cell carcinoma (28), adenoid cystic carcinoma (2), mucoepidermoid carcinoma (2), carcinosarcoma (1) and osteosarcoma (1). The sites of the cancer were tongue (7), tonsil (5), parotid (5), nasopharynx (3), soft and hard palate (3), larynx (2), base of tongue (2), oropharynx (2), buccal mucosa (1), maxilla (2), ear (1) and submandibular gland (1).

There are various conventions for referring to mouth, head and neck cancers, which is hardly surprising when you look at the list of sites in that last paragraph. In the title we use the all-inclusive mouth, head and neck cancers, but we're the first to admit that it's awkward and takes up a lot of space on the page. Some of the contributors have referred to mouth cancer, others to head and neck cancer and then there are the loyal souls who used the whole nine yards of it, and even use the plural at the end. We have allowed the variations, because we trust you to know what we're talking about in every instance.

Structure of this book

We have put a list of some of the terms you might not have come across before at the start of the book in a section called **Medical Terms**. This is for reference and is meant to be helpful. Please don't be put off by it. You can skip over it until you need an explanation for a particular term, or you may not need it at all.

Part One, *What To Expect From Treatment* contains a series of short pieces written by professionals involved in the care of mouth, head and neck cancer patients. Each has written an overview of what a person in treatment might expect, based on their perspective and expertise, always allowing for the spectrum of individual responses to treatment. Again, we stress that even if thirty people have had a particular experience, that does not necessarily mean you will.

This section also contains brief descriptions of complementary therapies which some people have found helpful and a more detailed account of yoga written by Anne L'Hénoret, one of our contributors who is also a yoga teacher.

Part Two, *Personal Accounts* is a collection of memoirs written by people who have experienced the disease and its treatment, and covers a range of situations and issues which arose for the contributors. These issues may or may not affect you. Contributors have offered insights and solutions that worked for them. These recommendations are included here as a guide only. We do not endorse any particular solutions. Some are common sense, but what works for one person does not necessarily work for everyone. If, at any stage during your treatment, you encounter difficulties, you should talk to your medical team.

Part Three, *Food, Eating and Recipes* offers some basic approaches to food and recipes that our contributors liked and found easy to prepare.

Part Four, *Resources and Contacts* lists books, CDs and websites that you may find helpful, and also contains a list of useful contacts. It is as current and comprehensive as we could make it when we went to print.

Finally, the **Index** at the back of the book is designed to help you find particular topics with ease. Once your treatment is underway, you may or may not find yourself challenged by side effects. If you do, for example, experience dry mouth due to a reduction in saliva, or general anxiety, or pain, or even something like claustrophobia in the context of lying still when surrounded by medical equipment – go to the Index, where you'll find an alphabetical list of topics covered, with page numbers where you will find the relevant entries.

Word of Mouth: Coping with and Surviving Mouth, Head and Neck Cancers is a non-commercial publication and is not for sale. Our goal is to make the book as widely available as possible, as a free download from the Dublin Dental University Hospital website (www.dentalhospital.ie), as a free e-book, and as a printed book.

Denise MacCarthy and Lia Mills

————◆————

MEDICAL TERMS: *Words You May Need to Know*

3-Dimensional conformal (3-DCRT): A technique using 3D images to plan and deliver the dose of radiation to the tumour

Acupuncture: Acupuncture is a complementary medical practice that entails stimulating certain points on the body, most often by penetrating the skin with a needle, to alleviate pain or to treat various diseases

Adenoid cystic carcinoma (ACC): This is an uncommon form of malignant neoplasm occurring most commonly in the major and minor salivary glands of the head and neck

Administration staff: Staff in hospitals and medical practices who organise appointments and provide information

Alopecia: Abnormal loss of hair, a common side effect of chemotherapy

Auriculotemporal nerve: A parasympathetic nerve associated with the parotid salivary gland

Bell's palsy: See facial nerve

Benign: Non-malignant; non-cancerous

Biopsy: A sample of cells taken from tissue where a problem is suspected. These cells are later examined under a microscope in the laboratory to see if any cancer cells are present

Bisphosphonate-related osteonecrosis of the jaws (BRONJ): Chemonecrosis of the jaws associated with the use of high-dose bisphosphonate therapy in certain forms of cancer

Brachytherapy: The practice of implanting radioactive material directly into or near a tumour

Carcinosarcoma: A malignant tumour that is a mixture of carcinoma (cancer of epithelial tissue, which is skin and tissue that lines or covers the internal organs) and sarcoma (cancer of connective tissue, such as bone, cartilage and fat)

Chemonecrosis: The death of cells and body parts caused by a chemical agent

Chemo-radiotherapy: Radiotherapy and chemotherapy combined to cure or control cancer

Chemotherapy: The use of drugs to cure or control cancer

Chest X-ray: An X-ray often performed before an operation to check the condition of the lungs. It is especially useful if someone has a history of smoking

Chlorhexidine: A chemical used to control oral bacteria and infection

Clinical nurse specialist: Qualified nurses who have additional training and qualifications in a specialised area of nursing practice

Cognitive behaviour therapy (CBT): An evidence based therapy that examines all elements that maintain a problem, including our thoughts (cognitions), feelings, behaviour and the environment. It is a structured therapy, which involves a partnership between you and your therapist

Computed tomography scan (CT scan): A scan used to diagnose disease or to determine where radiation needs to be delivered

Counsellor: See psychologist

Craniofacial surgery: Subspecialty of plastic surgery and oral and maxillofacial surgery that aims to treat and normalise deformities of the skull, face and jaws, whether congenital or acquired

CT neck and thorax/chest: A detailed scan in which a 'dye' can be injected into a vein to help see and build up a detailed picture of the tissues inside your body. You lie very still while you pass through the CT machine (which looks a bit like a giant doughnut). The scan takes approximately 15 to 30 minutes to complete

CT scan: See computed tomography scan

Dental hygienist: A dental professional who is qualified to provide oral hygiene advice and to carry out scaling of the teeth and preventive therapy

Dental implants: Titanium inserts placed in the jaw to help retain prosthetic appliances such as dentures. Implants are also used to retain ear, eye and nose prostheses

Dental obturator: A prosthetic device used to restore function following acquired defects of the palate that are the result of the surgical treatment of cancer

Dental specialist: Also called a dental oncologist. This is a dentist who performs pre-radiotherapy dental and oral assessments and provides long-term care to mouth, head and neck cancer patients

Dietitian: A health professional who is qualified to give accurate advice and information on all aspects of nutrition and diet

Dry mouth (Xerostomia): Side effect of radiotherapy if the saliva glands are affected by the radiation

Dysarthria: Slurred speech

Dysphagia: Difficulty swallowing

Dysphonia: Hoarseness

Electro cardiogram (ECG): A tracing of the heart to make sure it is beating in a regular way, often necessary before an operation

Endodontist: A dentist who specialises in the treatment of non-vital teeth

ENT: Ear, nose and throat

ENT surgeon: A surgeon who specialises in treating conditions of the ear, nose, throat, head and neck

Erythema: Redness/irritation of the skin during radiotherapy treatment

EUA: Examination under an anaesthetic to determine the extent of the disease. You are 'put to sleep' in theatre and the surgeon can then have a look in your throat, mouth and sinus area without causing you pain

External beam radiotherapy: Radiation beam from outside the body, directed at the tumour

Facial nerve (seventh cranial nerve): The facial nerve controls the movement of the muscles of the face. It passes through the parotid gland and has five branches going to different areas of the face and neck. Bell's palsy is weakness in your facial muscles which makes half of your face appear to droop. It may happen gradually or suddenly. This can affect your ability to smile or close your eye. The exact cause is unknown, but it may be the result of a viral infection of the facial nerve. Symptoms usually start to improve within a few weeks, with complete recovery taking about six months. Facial paralysis may be a side effect of surgery to the parotid gland or the neck. This is usually permanent if the nerve has been cut

Fibre-optic endoscopic examination of swallowing (FEES): Examination of swallowing, viewed via an endoscope (camera) passed through the nose while the patient attempts to swallow food and/or fluids

Fine needle aspirate (FNA): The removal of a few cells for analysis from the 'lump' using a needle and syringe. It is not a sore procedure, but it does sting a little when the needle goes in

Fluoride: Fluoride is a naturally occurring element. It is scientifically proven to remineralise teeth affected by decay. In Ireland, fluoride is generally available in our tap water and also in fluoridated toothpaste. When you are at a high risk of decay, application of more concentrated fluoride is advisable

Frey's syndrome: Frey's syndrome is caused by surgical injury to a nerve (the auriculotemporal nerve) that signals the salivary glands to secrete saliva. During the healing process the nerve regenerates and reattaches to sweat glands in the face instead of the original salivary gland (which was removed during surgery). Now when the patient eats the signal that should be going to the salivary gland travels to its new connection on the sweat glands and the patient experiences facial sweating and redness (salivaryglandforum.com)

GDP: General dental practitioner

GP: General medical practitioner

Gray (Gy): The international system (SI) unit of radiation dose expressed in terms of absorbed energy per unit mass of tissue. The gray is the unit of absorbed dose and has replaced the rad. 1 gray = 1 joule/kilogramme and also = 100 rad

Humidification: Air is normally warmed and moisturised as it passes through the nose and mouth. If you have a tracheostomy or a very dry mouth, a humidifier will be helpful to moisturise the air, especially at nighttime

ICU: Intensive care unit

IMRT: Intensity-modulated radiation therapy (IMRT) is an advanced type of radiation therapy used to treat cancer and non-cancerous tumours. IMRT uses advanced technology to manipulate beams of radiation to conform to the shape of a tumour. IMRT uses multiple small radiation beams of varying intensities to precisely radiate a tumour. The radiation intensity of each beam is controlled, and the beam shape changes throughout each treatment. The goal of IMRT is to bend the radiation dose to avoid or reduce exposure of healthy tissue and limit the side effects of treatment (Mayo Clinic)

Laryngectomy: The surgical removal of the larynx (voice box), resulting in voice loss and permanent neck breathing

Larynx: The voice box, located at your Adam's apple, containing your vocal cords, which produce voice

Leukoplakia: A white patch on the surface of the mucous membrane of the mouth that cannot be rubbed off

Lichen planus: Chronic mucocutaneous disease that affects the skin, tongue and oral mucosa. The underlying pathology is currently unknown

Linear accelerator: A machine used by a radiation therapist to deliver radiation

Magnetic resonance imaging (MRI) scan: This scan uses magnetic imaging to build up a picture of the tissues of whichever part of your body is being scanned. It is a very noisy scan but not painful. The doctor will inject a dye into your arm before the scan

Malignant: A growth or lump is said to be malignant when it is found to be cancerous. It can spread both locally and to distant parts of the body (metastasis)

Mask or immobilisation device: Keeps patient in the correct and reproducible position for each radiotherapy treatment

Maxillofacial prosthodontist: A dentist who specialises in the provision of prostheses, including dentures and obturators to replace parts of the jaw removed due to cancer

Maxillofacial surgeon: A surgeon trained in the treatment of diseases of the head, neck, face, mouth and jaws and their re-construction

Medical oncologist: A doctor who specialises in treating cancer patients using chemotherapy or biological therapies

Medical social worker: A professional who works with patients and their families in need of psychosocial help

Metastasis: The spread of cancer from one part of your body to another part

MHNC: Mouth, head and neck cancer

Mindfulness: The act of being intensely aware of what you're sensing and feeling at every moment, without interpretation or judgment. Awareness turned inward toward present felt experience

MLB (microlaryngobronchoscopy): A procedure in which the surgeon examines your larynx (voice box) and the upper part of your windpipe when you are asleep under an anaesthetic

MMUH: Mater Misericordiae University Hospital

Mould room: Where the mould and mask for radiation therapy are made

Mucoepidermoid carcinoma: Common salivary gland neoplasm, accounting for approximately 35 per cent of all malignancies of the major and minor salivary glands. They may contain squamous cells, mucus-secreting cells, and 'intermediate' cells

Mucositis: Inflammation and ulceration of the mucous membrane (skin/lining) of the mouth and throat during radio and chemotherapy

Naso-gastric tube (NGT): A thin tube that is passed through the nose and down into the stomach. It is used for giving special liquid food, drugs and fluids to patients who are unable to take adequate amounts by mouth in the short term

Nebuliser: A machine that converts liquid medication into a fine mist that can then be inhaled (Asthma Foundation)

Nutrition: Eating a wide variety of foods to ensure your body gets the energy and nutrition needed for growth and repair

Nutrition, artificial support: See percutaneous endoscopic gastrostomy (PEG); Naso-gastric tube (NGT)

Obturator: See dental obturator

Occupational therapist: A professional trained to use treatments which develop, recover, or maintain the daily living and work skills of patients

Oesophageal dilation: A procedure that allows your doctor to dilate, or stretch, a narrowed area of your oesophagus (swallowing tube)

OPG: Orthopantogram or panorex. This is a jaw X-ray. It is useful to check the condition of the teeth and also sometimes to make sure that the bone is not invaded by the tumour or in some cases broken

Oral surgeon: A speciality of dentistry, involving hard- and soft-tissue surgery of the mouth and jaws

Osteo-radionecrosis (ORN): The jawbone is affected by radiation treatment and may develop osteo-radionecrosis, which can result in a serious and severe infection and non-healing after trauma such as a dental extraction

Osteosarcoma: Malignant tumour of bone which is the eighth most common tumour of childhood

Panendoscopy and biopsy: The examination by a surgeon of your mouth, nose, throat, pharynx (back of throat), larynx (voice box), trachea (windpipe) and oesophagus (feeding pipe) when you are asleep under anaesthetic

Passy-Muir Speaking Valve: A speaking valve fitted to a tracheostomy tube to help speech production (if the vocal cords are not removed)

Pathologist: A medical doctor based in a laboratory who examines the histological (cellular) structure of diseased tissue removed by the surgeon, and confirms the diagnosis

Percutaneous endoscopic gastrostomy (PEG): A small tube which is passed endoscopically into your stomach through your abdominal wall. It is used for giving specialised liquid foods, drugs and fluids to patients who are anticipated to be unable to take adequate amounts by mouth in the long term, i.e. longer than two months

Periodontist: A dentist who specialises in the treatment of periodontal or gum disease

Physiotherapy and physiotherapist: Physiotherapists help to return muscle and body movement and function that has been lost through injury, surgery or the effects of surgery

Pilates: A body-conditioning practice that may help to build flexibility, muscle strength, and endurance in the legs, abdominals, arms, hips and back

Plastic surgeon: A medical specialist who deals with reconstructive and micro-vascular surgery. This is a technically difficult area and is important for placement of free flaps which are vital to reconstruct tissue and structures that have been surgically removed

Positron emission tomography scan (PET Scan or PET CT): This is a very useful scan to gain more detailed information about the cancer in your body. It uses a low dose of radioactive sugar to measure the activity within cells. You may have to go on a special low sugar/carbohydrate diet the day before the scan. You will be given instructions from the PET Scan Department if this is the case

Psychologist: A professional who is trained to evaluate, diagnose, treat, and study behaviour and mental processes. Clinical and counselling psychologists provide mental healthcare

Radiation oncologist: A doctor who specialises in treating cancer patients with radiation

Radiation stent: A plastic device to hold the jaws apart and move tissue (e.g. the tongue) out of the radiation field. This helps to protect healthy tissue from the effects of radiation

Radiation therapist: A professional who provides information on and delivers the radiation treatment

Radiographer: A professional trained to take radiographs and other types of scans such as CT and MRI

Radiologist: A medical specialist qualified to prescribe and interpret radiographs

Radiotherapy: See brachytherapy, external beam radiotherapy and IMRT

Reiki: A Japanese complementary therapy

Saliva: Saliva moisturises and protects the mouth. It contains enzymes that help digest food. It also contains antibodies that help protect against infections of the mouth and throat.

Salivary glands: Glands that produce saliva and deliver it into the mouth. They are called parotid, submandibular, sublingual and minor salivary glands. The glands are usually present in pairs, one at each side of the mouth.

Secretions: A build-up of mucous in your mouth, throat or larynx (airway), which may be difficult to remove following surgery if you cannot cough

Secretion suction machine: Mechanical device to suck out phlegm/mucous from the mouth, throat or larynx (airway), or through the laryngectomy

SIVH: South Infirmary Victoria Hospital, Cork

Speech and language therapy/therapist (SLT): A speech and language therapist assesses and provides therapy for speech, voice and swallowing disorders

Squamous cell carcinoma: A malignant tumour of the epithelium or lining tissue. It is the most common form of malignancy in mouth, head and neck cancers

Staging: The staging of a cancer describes its size and whether it has spread to other parts of the body

Tai chi: Also called tai chi chuan, this is a non-competitive, self-paced system of gentle physical exercise and stretching

TheraBite: The TheraBite Jaw Motion Rehabilitation System is a portable system specifically designed to treat reduced jaw opening

Thrush: A fungal infection which presents as white patches in the mouth. It is treated with antifungals

Tinnitus: Noise or ringing in the ears. Tinnitus isn't a condition itself — it's a symptom of an underlying condition, such as age-related hearing loss, ear injury or a circulatory system disorder

Tracheostomy: An opening that is made through the skin in the front of the neck into the trachea (windpipe). A tracheostomy tube is inserted into this opening to assist your breathing. This is necessary following a laryngectomy and is permanent. It may also be done following surgery when the mouth or throat are too sore and swollen to breath normally. In this instance the tube is usually removed when the swelling reduces. A tracheostomy nurse manages the tracheostomy and advises the patient about long-term care

Trismus: Difficulty opening the mouth

Ultrasound scan: In this scan a picture is built up of tissues using sound waves. This test is not painful and takes only 10 to 15 minutes to complete

Videofluoroscopy: An examination of the actual swallowing mechanism under X-ray surveillance and to access the possible aspiration (fluids/food going into the airway

Vocal cords: Muscles in the larynx (voice box) that help produce voice and sound

Voice prosthesis: A silicone device used after laryngectomy (removal of the voice box) to help restore voice and speech production

Xerostomia: see dry mouth

Yankauer suction tip: This is a firm plastic suction tip with a bulbous head that allows suction to take place without damaging surrounding structures. It is very useful to clear secretions from the tracheostomy site

Yoga: This is a generic term for the physical, mental and spiritual practices that originated in ancient India with the goal to attain a state of permanent peace. Modern-day yoga practitioners report musculoskeletal and mental health improvements. Yoga practice has been shown to improve mood and help with anxiety more than other metabolically matched exercises. Yoga is used with cancer patients to decrease depression, insomnia, pain and fatigue, and to increase anxiety control

Maxilla (upper jaw)

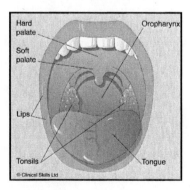

Mandible (lower jaw)

Nasopharynx

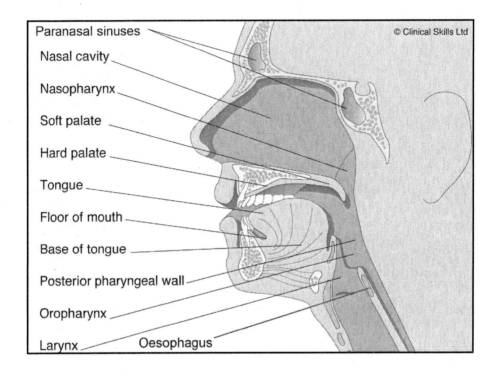

© Clinical Skills Ltd

Paranasal sinuses

Nasal cavity

Nasopharynx

Soft palate

Hard palate

Tongue

Floor of mouth

Base of tongue

Posterior pharyngeal wall

Oropharynx

Larynx

Oesophagus

The Salivary Glands

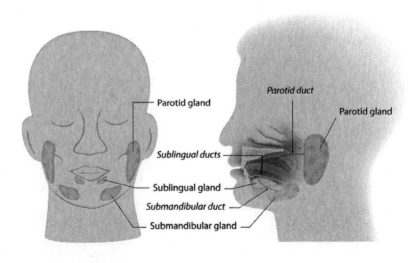

Parotid duct

Parotid gland

Parotid gland

Sublingual ducts

Sublingual gland

Submandibular duct

Submandibular gland

TREATMENT PATHWAY FOR
MOUTH, HEAD AND NECK CANCER

Concerned individual attends general medical (GP) or dental (GDP) practitioner

REFERRED TO SURGEON FOR INVESTIGATION
Ear, nose and throat (ENT) or maxillofacial surgeon

Radiologist

Radiographer

(radiographs and scans)

Biopsy of tissue, routine
examination, blood tests

Pathologist

(histopathological exam)

Multidisciplinary team (MDT) meeting

DISCUSSON, DIAGNOSIS AND TREATMENT PLAN

In attendance: surgeon(s), radiologist, pathologist, radiation oncologist, medical
oncologist, dentist, speech therapist, radiographer, specialist nurses in surgery and
chemotherapy, tracheostomy nurse, physiotherapist, dietitian

IMMEDIATE TREATMENT

Following MDT planning, the proposed treatment is discussed with the patient and
their family and supporters

Treatment may involve one or combinations of surgery, radiotherapy, chemotherapy
and palliative care

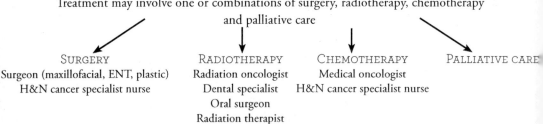

SURGERY	RADIOTHERAPY	CHEMOTHERAPY	PALLIATIVE CARE
Surgeon (maxillofacial, ENT, plastic)	Radiation oncologist	Medical oncologist	
H&N cancer specialist nurse	Dental specialist	H&N cancer specialist nurse	
	Oral surgeon		
	Radiation therapist		
	Mould room/mask		

IMMEDIATE AND LONG-TERM CARE

Follow-up is an important part of treatment and will be provided by your speech
therapist, tracheostomy nurse, dietitian, physiotherapist, occupational therapist,
surgeon(s), radiologist, pathologist, radiation oncologist, medical oncologist, specialist
nurses, dentist, maxillofacial prosthodontist, dental hygienist, oral surgeon, psycho-
oncologist, psychiatrist, counsellor and medical social worker

PART ONE

What to Expect from Treatment

Advice from the professionals

INTRODUCTION

A large team of people will be involved in your referral, assessment, diagnosis, treatment, rehabilitation and long-term support following a diagnosis of mouth, head and neck cancer. Your journey will start with your general medical or dental practitioner, and then a referral to a maxillofacial or ear, nose and throat (ENT) surgeon, plastic surgeon, medical oncologist, radiation oncologist, pathologist, tracheostomy nurse, radiologist, clinical nurse specialist, administration staff, radiation therapist, dental specialist, dental hygienist, oral surgeon, speech therapist, physiotherapist, dietitian occupational therapist, maxillofacial prosthodontist, medical social worker, psychologist and counsellor. The roles of the maxillofacial or ENT surgeon, medical oncologist and radiation oncologist will be very clear from the start of your treatment and you will form a strong relationship with these individuals. However, there is a team of professionals whose input will be essential to your ongoing well-being and rehabilitation. Their contributions are presented in this section.

THE PATIENT JOURNEY

Margaret McGrath, Head and Neck Cancer Nurse
Co-ordinator, Mater Misericordiae University Hospital, Dublin

So your doctor or dentist has referred you to an ENT or maxillofacial surgeon ...

Maybe you have found a lump, have a non-healing mouth ulcer, are hoarse, have developed swallow problems, have pain – there are many reasons why your GP or dentist might refer you to an ENT or maxillofacial surgeon. In this short summary I will attempt to explain what you might experience. I am basing this on over 14 years' experience of this very specialised area. As the majority (more than 80 per cent) of mouth, head and neck cancers we see in our clinics are squamous cell carcinomas (SCC) the following applies mainly to this type of cancer. However, most of the necessary tests and treatments will apply to other types also.

First visit to the clinic

The surgeon will take a history from you, asking questions like, *How long have you had this problem? When did you first notice this lump/ulcer? Do you smoke? Do you drink alcohol? Have you noticed any problems with swallow?* She or he will then do an examination, including a neck examination (feel your neck), and perhaps put a scope (fine tube) down your throat (not nearly as bad as it sounds). If you have a sore in your mouth, she or he might take a tiny piece of it away (a biopsy) and send it to the pathology laboratory for histological examination (analysis). It is likely that you might even need to be admitted for a biopsy and perhaps some scans and investigations. Now that you have worked up the courage to come and see us, it is best to keep the investigations moving so we find out what the matter is and get you sorted and well again. Necessary investigations may include some or all of the following. (See Medical Terms for more information.)

➤ Chest X-ray

➤ Ultrasound of the neck

➤ CT Mouth, Neck and Chest or PET/CT Scan

➤ MRI scan of the head and neck area

➤ Fine needle aspiration of the lump (FNA)

➤ Jaw X-ray (OPG)

➤ Routine blood tests

➤ An ECG may be appropriate before you go to theatre for a biopsy

➤ Panendoscopy and biopsy (examination of the mouth/nose/throat/sinus area when you are in theatre)

➤ Microlaryngobronchoscopy (MLB)

➤ Examination under anaesthetic (EUA)

Once all the necessary tests are done, your surgeon will discuss your results at a multidisciplinary case conference (MDT). Here there will be several surgeons, a consultant pathologist, a consultant radiologist, a medical oncologist, a radiation oncologist, a specialist nurse and people from other disciplines. A provisional treatment plan will be suggested and then your doctor will discuss it with you (and a significant other if you wish) before deciding on the definite plan. We assess everyone's situation on an individual basis, so treatment plans can vary from one patient to another. However, your treatment plan will be devised based on standards of international and established best practice.

Staging

The stage and seriousness of the cancer can be determined using the following three factors:

T = size of tumour

N = presence or absence of cancer spread to the lymph nodes (glands) in your neck

M = spread of cancer to other areas of your body (metastasis or secondary cancer)

So we might grade a small tongue cancer as being a T1N0M0 (small primary tumour with no disease (cancer) in the lymph neck nodes and no disease anywhere else). This patient would most likely require surgery only. An example of a large tongue cancer might be a T3N2M0 cancer (big primary tongue tumour with disease (cancer) in the lymph nodes but no disease anywhere else). In these situations, a combination of treatments is likely to be required. Your surgical team will discuss your individual treatment plan in detail with you.

When the surgeon knows the stage of the cancer, it is then easier to plan the treatment.

Treatments

The specific treatment plan for you will take into account the following:

➤ Your age and general performance status (how healthy you are otherwise)

➤ The stage of your cancer based on the TNM stage above

➤ The expert opinions of the multidisciplinary team

➤ Your preference and opinion

Your surgeon will explain the treatment plan to you and tell you if she or he believes that the treatment can cure or control the disease. The main treatments (often combinations) we use are:

➤ Surgery

➤ Radiotherapy

➤ Chemotherapy

- ➤ Biological Therapies
- ➤ Palliative Care

You may need one or two or even three of these treatments.

Surgery

Surgery is still one of the main treatments for mouth, head and neck cancer. Usually the smaller the tumour, the smaller the surgery required. The aim of the surgery is to remove all the cancer cells/tumour with a margin of healthy cells. Sometimes skin, muscle, lymph gland and bone need to be removed during the surgery. The surgeon may need to take skin, muscle and/or bone from somewhere else to reconstruct the area after the tumour is removed; this is called reconstruction.

Both your function, i.e. how you eat, drink, talk, breathe, and your appearance are very important to us after your operation. If part of your palate has been removed you may need an obturator. This is usually a plastic extension of a normal denture that replaces the part of the jaw that was removed during surgery.

When the surgery is extensive, the first week afterwards may be especially tough. You may need to be in intensive care or the high-dependency unit (HDU). You may be fed through a feeding tube, and you might even need a special breathing tube (tracheostomy), but hang in there as best you can, as you will start to feel better once you are over the first week. Do let the surgeon and other team members know how you are feeling, especially if you feel like you are struggling in those early days after surgery. We are all here to help you get through this very difficult time.

Radiotherapy

Radiotherapy is the use of special X-rays to kill or sometimes shrink the cancer cells/tumour. Sometimes radiotherapy is the main (primary) treatment and sometimes it is used after surgery. Normally radiotherapy is given over a period of five to seven weeks. You have it each day Monday to Friday and each treatment lasts approximately ten minutes. Most patients tell me that it is not too bad for the first two to three weeks but that the side effects (pain, red skin, tiredness, dry mouth, worsening swallow) can start to become more troublesome from week three to four. But don't forget, time passes no matter what and this time will pass too. Just remember not to suffer in silence and let your doctor, nurse or therapist know if you have any pain or if you have difficulty with keeping your weight up.

Chemotherapy

Chemotherapy is the use of drugs to kill or control cancer cells. Sometimes it is given before and during radiotherapy. Sometimes it is given before surgery and sometimes it is given three to six times during the six to seven weeks of radiotherapy. It is thought that having chemotherapy in conjunction with radiotherapy for squamous cell carcinoma (SCC) may help the radiotherapy to work better. If you get chemotherapy as well as radiotherapy you must be especially good with your oral healthcare as you will be even more prone to getting a sore mouth. Also tiredness may be more of a bother, but do persevere as the chemotherapy usually ends when the radiotherapy ends, after six to seven weeks of treatment.

Biological therapies

Some patients will be unable to tolerate chemotherapy and we might then consider using a biological treatment. These drugs are sometimes called targeted therapies. With this treatment drugs use your body's own immune system to fight the cancer. They are usually given with radiotherapy once a week, or sometimes on their own.

Palliative care

Our colleagues in palliative care are specialists in pain and symptom management. Sometimes patients with mouth, head and neck cancer can experience a type of pain that we call neuropathic, or nerve, pain. Here our palliative care teams are a great help. They also help when we have patients with very aggressive cancers that we cannot cure. For these patients we do our very best to control the symptoms, especially pain.

The palliative care team is a great help when it comes to getting patients home, as they have colleagues working in the community who visit patients in their own homes and make sure that their quality of life is as good as possible for as long as possible. Sometimes a patient may need their help for only a short time after treatment, especially if you go home on very strong painkillers such as morphine, and sometimes patients and their families need their help for longer.

What happens after the treatment is finished

In the mouth, head and neck cancer centre where I work, we follow up our patients very closely after their cancer treatments. In the first year, you might be seen every six to eight weeks depending on how you are and what treatment you received. We sometimes use scans to help us monitor how effective the treatment has been. If appropriate these might be done three months after the radiotherapy is completed. Sometimes, especially as time goes by, it is sufficient for the surgeon to examine your mouth and throat, do a scope and feel your neck. If she or he is worried about anything you may be booked in for a biopsy just to be sure that all is well.

Other people working in our clinic include a dietitian, a speech and language therapist and an audiologist, and you may see one or more of these specialists at some stage during your recovery.

As time passes, the gap between appointments usually gets longer. Depending on the type of cancer, after five years of monitoring, we can sometimes discharge a patient to their GP. Some patients prefer to come back to us even once a year after that time just to be sure. Of course if a patient is worried she or he can always contact our team and they will be seen in the next clinic if at all possible.

Conclusion

As an oncology nurse who has worked with patients with cancer for more than 25 years, I will be the first to acknowledge that mouth, head and neck cancer is a very difficult disease. At times the treatments may appear worse than the illness itself. We may ask some of you to completely change your lifestyle (stop smoking and/or drinking alcohol). Some of you may well have to learn to swallow or speak again. Some of you will require a PEG feeding tube (a tube that is inserted directly into the stomach for feeding) or even a tracheostomy (breathing) tube. Those of us working in this area acknowledge that life will be both different and difficult for you for a period. My patients tell me that the battle is often to keep strong and carry on, as this hard time too will pass.

I have enjoyed reading the patients' stories, as these people are the real experts. I have had the great pleasure of knowing some of these patients and I remember how they struggled as we all would in the early days. It is great to read how life is for them now. I know that you will find this book helpful and I applaud the Dublin Dental University Hospital for supporting and producing it. I also thank our mouth, head and neck cancer patients for managing to inspire me on a daily basis.

———•———

RADIOTHERAPY

Agnella Craig, Assistant Professor, Discipline of Radiation Therapy, School of Medicine, Trinity College Dublin

What is radiotherapy?

Radiotherapy is the use of high-energy X-rays to treat and cure cancer or to relieve a patient's symptoms. Radiotherapy works by destroying the cancer cells. Radiation can come from outside the body (external beam radiotherapy) or a small container of radioactive material can be implanted in the body, directly into or near the tumour (brachytherapy). Some patients receive both kinds of radiotherapy, but most patients with tumours in the head and neck region will have external beam radiotherapy.

Radiotherapy can be used after surgery (post-operative), with other treatments such as chemotherapy (chemo-radiation) or it can be used before surgery to reduce the size of a tumour to be operated on. Your doctor will tell you what the best approach is for your situation, taking all the relevant factors into account.

The radiation oncologist is the specialist doctor who prescribes radiotherapy, makes decisions on what area of the body should be treated, and on what the best method of delivery is.

The approach used can be either 3-DCRT (3-dimensional conformal radiotherapy) or IMRT (intensity modulated radiotherapy). 3-DCRT involves shaping the dose to match the shape of the tumour. This allows a high dose to be directed at the tumour while sparing the normal tissue as much as possible. IMRT is a more complex technique that allows the intensity of the dose to change around the tumour and keeps the dose to normal tissues very low. IMRT requires a longer planning stage and longer treatment delivery times (how long you lie on the bed every day to have treatment). Nowadays IMRT is used commonly, but sometimes a similar plan can be created using the 3-DCRT approach without the long treatment delivery times.

External beam radiotherapy is usually given five days a week, Monday to Friday. A course of treatment will usually last seven to eight weeks. You will be in the treatment room for between ten and 30 minutes depending on how many sections/angles your treatment is divided into.

The radiation therapist is one of the main contact people for you during your treatment. She or he will give you information on the treatment procedure and will also carry out the treatment using a machine called a linear accelerator.

What to expect

Before your radiotherapy starts, you may need to visit the dentist to check the condition of your teeth and gums. The radiation oncologist will organise this appointment for you.

The first step in the radiotherapy department is to have an immobilisation device made. This is called a mask/shell/cast/Orfit. This mask has two functions:

> ➤ It keeps you in the correct position so the treatment can be targeted accurately

> ➤ The area to be treated can be marked out on the mask rather than putting marks on your face or neck

You will wear your mask each time you come for treatment. It only takes a short while to have a mask made and the radiation therapist will explain everything to you beforehand.

The next step is a CT scan, which will usually happen on the same day as the mask is made. The CT scan is used to show exactly where the treatment needs to be directed. This is usually the tumour, a small area around the tumour and some lymph nodes, or if you have had surgery, it is the area from which the tumour was removed.

Once this scan is taken and some marks are put on your mask, you can return home while work begins on creating your treatment plan.

Using your scan, the radiation oncologist will highlight the treatment area and a plan will be designed to treat the tumour with a high dose and keep the dose to normal tissues as low as possible.

On your first day of treatment, the procedure will be fully explained to you. You will also be given information about side effects and advice on how to minimise these. You can bring a pen and paper with you to make notes or have someone with you to listen to this information.

As the radiotherapy has to be delivered to the same area every day, some quality assurance checks are carried out while you receive treatment. These include taking regular images (special X-rays or CT scans) when you are in the treatment room, to check your position and the area treated. The radiation therapists will be in the room with you at the start, to set up the equipment. Once the treatment is ready, they will leave the room to switch on the machine. They can hear and see you at all times from outside the room. You will hear noises from the machine and it may move around you. It will not touch you and you will not feel anything. It is just like having an X-ray taken, only it takes longer.

Side effects

Like all forms of cancer treatment, radiotherapy has side effects. The side effects will depend on many factors, including the area being treated, whether you are having other treatments such as chemotherapy, and the radiotherapy approach. Some side effects will occur during your treatment and last for a short while after treatment finishes, but some might be permanent. Your radiation oncologist will describe the side effects you might experience before you start treatment. Possible side effects include:

➤ Skin reaction. Redness/irritation called erythema
  - *Be careful when washing and shaving. Use only the creams recommended*

➤ Tiredness, fatigue
  - *Get rest but also take some gentle exercise, daily if possible*

➤ Temporary or permanent hair loss in the treated area

➤ Sore mouth (mucositis). If not managed correctly, this may lead to infections such as thrush
  - *Keep your mouth clean. Use the recommended mouthwashes, e.g. bread soda and water solution*

➤ Pain/difficulty in eating and swallowing. This can lead to weight loss
  - *Stick to soft foods. Avoid anything hard, sharp, too hot or too cold. Try to eat little and often rather than having three meals a day. Take your time when eating. If eating is painful, take your pain medications a set time before your meal to get maximum relief*

➤ Dry mouth (Xerostomia)
  - *Carry a water bottle everywhere and sip from it as often as you can. Keep a glass of water beside your bed. Use saliva substitutes as recommended by the dental team*

➤ Distorted sense of taste
  - *Try foods you didn't like before, but accept that everything might be tasteless for a while*

➤ Hoarseness or a change in the sound of your voice

Do's and Don'ts

Do:

➤ Make sure you get all the information you need to help you through this. If you don't understand something, ask questions!

➤ Talk to your radiation therapist. Let her/him know what is going on. Report any changes you notice. Some changes are expected and normal but the staff can give you advice on how to manage these

➤ If you talk to other patients about their experience, remember your cancer and experience will probably be different from theirs

➤ Always take the advice of your dietitian, dental team and speech and language therapist

➤ Give up the fags, or cut down. Smoking will make the side effects worse. Nicotine replacement therapy can help

Don't:

➤ Never use creams such as Sudocrem on your skin while having radiotherapy. Only use the recommended products

➤ If you become hoarse, don't force your voice. Give it time to recover

➤ Drink fluids. Stay well hydrated even if it is difficult to swallow

➤ Try not to lose weight. If you do, make sure to let the RT know if your mask feels loose

➤ Don't miss a treatment appointment

————◆————

CHEMOTHERAPY

Therese Harvey, Medical Oncology Nurse Specialist,
St James's Hospital, Dublin

What is chemotherapy?

Chemotherapy is a treatment that uses drugs to cure or control cancer. These drugs can be injected into your bloodstream or given in tablet form. Chemotherapy may be used alone or in combination with another form of cancer treatment. It may be given at the same time as radiotherapy. This is called chemo-radiation. Sometimes chemotherapy is given to relieve symptoms and improve quality of life if it is not possible to cure the cancer. This is called palliative chemotherapy.

Chemotherapy drugs affect how a quickly cell divides and grows. They can affect normal cells as well as cancer cells, therefore side effects occur due to healthy cells being killed.

Biological therapies are drugs that come under the general umbrella of chemotherapy. They are also known as 'targeted therapies', as they are aimed directly at specific cells. Biological therapies use your body's immune system to fight cancer.

The medical oncologist is the doctor who specialises in treating cancer patients with chemotherapy and other drugs.

What to expect

Your case will be discussed at a multidisciplinary team meeting (MDT) to decide which is the best treatment for your cancer. In the majority of cases patients with head and neck cancers are referred to the medical oncologist by the surgeons (ENT or Maxillofacial) or by the radiation oncologist. Many patients find it daunting to have another team involved in their care, but the teams maintain close contact with each other.

If chemotherapy is to be considered as part of your treatment you will meet the medical oncologist and the specialist nurse to discuss treatment options. Your first meeting with the medical oncologist may be when you are still an inpatient recovering from surgery. At this time you may not be well enough for a decision to be made on your treatment plan. If this is the case an outpatient appointment will be made for you to finalise your treatment plan. This appointment will be for about two to three weeks later.

For many patients the first meeting with the medical oncologist will take place in the outpatient department. Before you arrive at this appointment you will have been informed by your surgeon or radiation oncologist that chemotherapy is a possible treatment for you.

Remember it is a good idea to take a family member or friend along to your appointment so someone else hears what the plan is.

Where is chemotherapy given?

Where you receive your chemotherapy will depend on your treatment plan. For some patients all chemotherapy is given in a chemotherapy day ward and will not require overnight admission. This may be given in your general hospital or in a specialist radiation oncology centre.

For other patients it will be necessary to spend some time as an inpatient, as the drugs may be given as infusions over a period of a few days.

Sometimes chemotherapy is administered via a slow infusion pump. This may be done at home over a few days.

You will hear the words *cycle* and *regimen* used in discussions about your chemotherapy treatment plan. These words refer to how many doses of chemotherapy you will receive and how often they will be given. Your medical oncologist and specialist nurse will discuss this with you in detail and give you written information on the drugs that will be used and the possible side effects.

If you have any questions about treatment ask your doctor or nurse at this visit. Some patients find it helpful to have a list of questions ready before coming to appointments. You will also have plenty of opportunity to discuss the chemotherapy with the nurses who administer your chemotherapy.

You will be given names and phone numbers of people to contact if you are unwell or if you have any concerns.

Before you receive chemotherapy you may be asked to sign a consent form saying that you have been informed of the risks and benefits of chemotherapy and of what side effects may occur.

The aim of chemotherapy is to either cure or control cancer but it is important to get the right balance of benefit versus risk. If at any stage you find coping with the treatment too difficult, discuss this with your medical oncologist or the nursing team. It may be necessary to change the treatment plan if you are not tolerating chemotherapy.

More scans may need to be carried out during treatment and a decision will be made whether to continue with the current treatment or to change the plan. You will be informed of any change to the plan and what the reason is for the change.

Your height and weight will be checked before your first chemotherapy treatment is given, as your chemotherapy dose is calculated according to the surface area of your body.

Before each cycle you will be reviewed by a doctor and your blood counts will be checked to ensure it is safe to go ahead with chemotherapy. Only after this will your chemotherapy infusion be made up. For this reason visits to the oncology day ward may take longer than you expect.

At times the doses may be adjusted to help lessen side effects. Sometimes it may be necessary to delay your treatment for a few days or weeks to allow you to recover from side effects.

A lot of chemotherapy is given via a drip. This will be given through a fine tube called a cannula, inserted into a vein, usually in the back of the hand. This will be taken out following each treatment and a new one inserted at each hospital visit.

For some chemotherapy regimens that require lengthy infusions of drugs it may be necessary to insert a more permanent tube to give chemotherapy through. The type most commonly used is called a peripherally inserted central catheter (PICC). This is a long thin flexible tube that is inserted into one of the large veins of the arm. This may stay in situ for months to allow chemotherapy to be infused over a number of treatments. It will be covered with a dressing and advice will be given to you on how to manage it when you are at home.

Another semi-permanent line that may be used is called a portocath or port. This is a device placed under your skin, generally on the chest wall, which is linked to a tube put into one of your veins. Some patients prefer this type of catheter, as it is not visible. However some hospitals may only use one type of catheter device.

POSSIBLE SIDE EFFECTS OF CHEMOTHERAPY AND WAYS TO PREVENT OR MANAGE THEM

Risk of infection

White blood cells help to fight infection. Chemotherapy can reduce the number of white blood cells. This is called neutropenia. Because of this you may become very unwell if infections are not treated quickly.

It is important to contact your doctor or nurse immediately if:

➤ Your temperature is 38° C or higher

➤ You feel unwell (with or without a temperature)

If you have a low white-blood-cell count and a high temperature you will need to be admitted to hospital for intravenous antibiotics

Bruising and bleeding

Platelets are blood cells that help the blood to clot. These may be reduced following chemotherapy. If you have any unexplained bruising or bleeding such as nosebleeds or bleeding gums, you need to inform your doctor or nurse. A blood test will show if your platelet count is low. A platelet transfusion may be required. This will generally be done as a day case.

Anaemia

Red cells are responsible for carrying oxygen around your body. If your red-cell count is low you may feel tired and breathless. Inform your doctor or nurse if this occurs. You may need a blood transfusion. This will also generally be done as a day case.

Feeling sick (nausea) and being sick (vomiting)

Anti-sickness medication is very effective now compared with what was available 20 years ago. You will be prescribed anti-sickness medication to prevent you being sick before you receive chemotherapy and for a few days following chemotherapy. It is important to take this as prescribed, as the risk of being sick from some chemotherapy drugs may last for a few days. If you still have nausea or vomiting despite taking anti-sickness medication, contact your doctor or nurse. It is important that you inform your team sooner rather than later as you may become dehydrated, as well as feeling miserable! Generally this side effect can be controlled by staying at home and taking different anti-sickness medication.

Steroids are often used as part of your anti-sickness medication. They can affect your sleep, so we generally recommend that they are taken early in the day.

Sore mouth

Before receiving chemotherapy you will have undergone a dental check. If required, extractions will be carried out before you start chemotherapy, as you are at increased risk of becoming unwell if you get gum infections when your blood count is reduced.

Your mouth may become sore or dry during treatment, especially if you are also receiving radiotherapy. You may also develop mouth ulcers. It is important to drink as much fluid as possible to keep your mouth moist, and to clean your mouth with a soft toothbrush. Many patients find it helps to suck ice. Mouthwashes may be prescribed at the start of chemotherapy, to prevent infection.

If you develop a sore or infected mouth it is important to inform your doctor or nurse, as mouthwashes and medication can be prescribed for this.

Diarrhoea

Some chemotherapy can cause diarrhoea. Contact your doctor or nurse if you have more than three loose bowel movements per day. It may be possible to control diarrhoea with oral medication. If you have diarrhoea it is important to drink lots of fluids. If diarrhoea does not settle you may have to attend hospital to receive fluids intravenously.

Constipation

Some chemotherapy (as well as anti-sickness and pain medication) may cause constipation. Contact your doctor or nurse if this occurs, as medication can be prescribed to treat it.

Changes in how you taste food

Some chemotherapy may cause foods to taste different. Some patients find it helps to add sauces and seasoning.

Hair loss

Some types of chemotherapy may cause your hair to fall out, whereas others may only cause thinning of hair. You will be informed if the drugs you are getting are likely to do this and you will be given advice about having a wig fitted if you wish. Some patients opt not to get a wig and decide to use scarves or hats. It is important to remember that your head will be more sensitive to heat and cold, so use hats and sunscreen to protect it.

Changes to hearing

Some chemotherapy may cause some hearing loss or ringing in the ears. Your hospital may routinely do a hearing check before starting chemotherapy. If you notice any hearing loss or ringing in your ears, tell your doctor or nurse. Your chemotherapy may be changed to a different type. Most patients find the ringing will eventually improve, but hearing loss may be permanent.

Heart side effects

Some drugs affect how your heart works. Inform your doctor or nurse if you feel any chest pain or tightness.

Skin changes

You skin colour may darken slightly following chemotherapy. During and following chemotherapy your skin will be more sensitive to the sun. It is important to cover up when exposed to the sun and to use high-factor sun-protection cream.

Some patients develop soreness and redness of the hands and feet. This is called hand-foot or plantar-palmer syndrome. Tell your doctor or nurse if you develop this. Wear loose-fitting socks or gloves and do not wear tight-fitting shoes. Use unperfumed soap and you will be advised on what moisturising cream to use.

Fertility

Some chemotherapy may affect your ability to become pregnant or to father a child. Your doctor or nurse will discuss this with you if chemotherapy drugs you are given have the potential to do this. If there is a risk that chemotherapy will cause permanent infertility you may wish to be referred to the HARI (Human Assisted Reproduction Ireland) unit in the Rotunda Hospital. Sperm banking or egg freezing may be an option for you.

Blood clots

Anyone who has cancer has an increased risk of developing a blood clot. If you are receiving chemotherapy this further increases the risk. If you notice any pain, swelling or redness in your leg or if you have breathlessness or chest pain, contact your doctor or nurse. If you develop a clot you can be treated with medication to thin your blood.

Specific side effects of biological therapies (targeted therapies)

These therapies may cause flu-like symptoms when they are first given. Apart from this the main side effects are rashes, tiredness and high blood pressure. If you develop a rash, creams will be prescribed to treat it.

ADDITIONAL INFORMATION

Contraception

It is not advisable to conceive or father a child while having chemotherapy, as the drugs used may harm your baby. A reliable barrier method of contraception, such as condoms, should be used when having chemotherapy and for a few months after.

Breastfeeding

Women are advised not to breastfeed while undergoing chemotherapy, as there is a possibility that chemotherapy drugs will be present in breast milk.

Other medication

Inform your doctor if you are taking any other medication before commencing chemotherapy. Do not take any herbal medication without checking with your doctor or nurse, as it may interact with your treatment.

Conclusion

It is important to remember that you can experience different side effects from someone else receiving the same chemotherapy as you.

Ask for advice from the medical and nursing team whenever you need it, and use any support available to you.

Keep your list of emergency contact numbers handy (in your phone, your bag or pinned to the fridge) so that you and your family have immediate access to expert advice.

If you need to be admitted to hospital for any reason, inform the doctor or nurse that you are receiving chemotherapy.

———•———

SPEECH AND SWALLOWING

Noreen O'Regan, B.Sc. Clin Lang, Senior Speech and Language Therapist, St James's Hospital, Dublin

Tumours of the head and neck usually involve the structures we use to talk and swallow. Hence the tumours themselves and the methods used to treat them often cause problems with talking, eating and drinking. Everybody's experience will be different but below are the changes most typically experienced.

SPEECH

Dysarthria (slurred speech)

This typically occurs with tumours of the lips, tongue, cheek, jaw and floor of the mouth.

The muscles in these areas, used for talking, are unable to move as quickly and accurately as they were before treatment, and so the speech they produce is slurred. The extent to which it is slurred varies depending on how restricted the movements are. It can range from mild slurring, where speech is less clear, to moderate slurring, where you often have to repeat what you say, to severe slurring, where you may be understood only by close family and friends who are used to hearing you.

Altered resonance (altered nasal speech tone)

This typically occurs with tumours of the tonsil, palate and maxilla (upper jaw).

These tissues control whether air comes through your mouth or nose when you talk. When they are not working fully your speech can sound nasal and be harder to understand. Sometimes a specialised denture called an obturator may be required to help this.

Dysphonia (hoarseness)

This typically occurs with tumours of the larynx (voice box) or with radiotherapy to the areas close by. If the muscles of the larynx or the vocal cords are swollen or unable to move as fully as before, the sound they make is hoarse. It may be mild (sounding like you have a sore throat) or more severe, where you have only a whispered voice and find it difficult to be heard.

Laryngectomy (permanent voice loss)

This typically occurs with larger tumours of the larynx that require it to be surgically removed. After this type of surgery you will have two main changes:

➤ You will have a permanent tracheostomy (see below) so that you breathe and cough through your neck

➤ You will lose the volume or sound of your voice completely

There are a number of options for replacing your voice:

➤ Voice prosthesis/speaking valve. The surgeon creates a small opening in your neck into which a silicone valve is fitted. Using your thumb (or a second valve) you can direct air through the valve to allow you to talk

➤ Electrolarynx. This is a battery operated electronic device that you hold against your neck or cheek when you talk. The device provides an electronic replacement for your voice

➤ Oesophageal speech. This method of talking, less frequently used recently, involves learning to swallow air into your gullet and regurgitate it (like we do when we burp), thereby producing sound for speech

Tracheostomy

This procedure is frequently completed at the time of surgery. It is required in the early days after surgery when the mouth or throat are too swollen to allow breathing through the mouth and nose. A tube is placed in the neck to allow breathing through the neck. Once the swelling reduces it is usually removed.

Because you breathe through the neck with this tube, air never reaches your mouth to allow you talk. Hence you can mouth words but no sound comes out. People typically communicate at this time via writing, texting and gesture. If writing is not an option, picture charts can be used to communicate. Once the tube is removed speech returns, with some of the changes outlined above.

SWALLOWING

Dysphagia (difficulty swallowing)

Dysphagia can occur with tumours in any part of the head and neck. It refers to difficulty eating, drinking and swallowing and may include the following symptoms:

In the mouth:

- ➤ Drooling
- ➤ Difficulty chewing, especially harder foods like meat
- ➤ Difficulty controlling and collecting food within your mouth. As a result food remains around your mouth after swallowing
- ➤ Difficulty moving food from the front of the mouth to the back for swallowing
- ➤ Nasal regurgitation – food and drink coming back down your nose

In the throat:

- ➤ Food or drink sticking in the throat and not travelling down to the oesophagus (gullet)
- ➤ Aspiration – food or drink going against your breath into your lungs instead of your oesophagus and stomach. This can lead to serious chest infections and pneumonia, as well as weight loss
- ➤ Weak cough. Just as your swallow can be weakened, so too can your cough, meaning you do not cough and splutter when food or drink goes down the wrong way

Typically, hard foods and liquids are the most difficult to swallow. Soft, moist or mashed foods like custard, rice pudding, thick soups, fish and shepherd's pie are usually easier. A modified diet may be recommended for you (e.g. a soft diet, a minced and moist diet or a smooth purée diet). Modified fluids (i.e. thickened to allow better, safer control of swallowing) may also be recommended. In more severe cases a feeding tube through the nose or stomach may be required to supplement or replace eating and drinking.

Xerostomia (dry mouth)

Dry mouth typically occurs when the salivary glands are removed in surgery or are affected by radiotherapy. It makes the mouth very dry and uncomfortable. It also makes swallowing difficult, as there is no moisture to mix through food as you chew or to help it move backwards in your mouth.

If it is safe for you to swallow, sipping fluids, particularly water, can help. So too can saliva substitutes and replacement gels (e.g. BioXtra). Adding lots of extra moisture to your food in the form of gravy, sauce, milk etc. can help. So too can taking fluids with your food. However, everybody is different and it is important to follow the advice you receive after your individual assessment.

Trismus (difficulty opening the mouth)

Surgery and radiotherapy can reduce the opening of your mouth, making eating, cleaning, talking and dental treatment difficult. With normal mouth opening you should be able to fit two and a half to three fingers between your teeth. If you have no teeth you should be able to fit four fingers between your jaws. If you notice this becoming more difficult you may need exercises to help stretch your mouth opening.

Timeframe

While every case is different, for most people these speech and swallowing difficulties occur as follows:

- ➤ **Surgery:** The problems develop straight after surgery, when they are at their worst, and improve gradually over the following weeks and months

- ➤ **Chemo/radiotherapy:** The problems develop gradually, in particular during the second half of treatment, and are at their most severe at the end of treatment and in the early weeks after it has finished. They then improve gradually in the weeks and months after treatment

- ➤ **Combined surgery and chemo/radiotherapy:** The problems develop after surgery and improve until the later weeks of radiotherapy when they deteriorate again. Improvement begins again in the weeks after treatment is completed.

Speech and language therapy (SLT)

Many people undergoing treatment for head and neck cancer will be referred by their doctor for speech and language therapy. This can occur before, during and after treatment and often involves:

➤ An information session before treatment begins to explain what changes you can expect

➤ Assessment of the structures and function of the mouth and throat for swallowing and talking. This typically includes:
  - *Examining the mouth and throat and its movements*
  - *Completing speech tasks (reading words and sentences aloud)*
  - *Evaluating control and swallowing of fluids and foods of various consistencies (e.g. water, yoghurt, bread)*
  - *Sometimes X-rays (videofluoroscopy) or camera tests of swallowing (FEES: fiberoptic endoscopic examination of swallowing) are required*

➤ Advising on the safest food and fluid consistencies to swallow. This is to minimise the risk of chest infections or pneumonia from aspiration

➤ Exercise programmes. These may be preventative and start before treatment, in the case of chemo/radiotherapy. In the case of surgery they usually begin once the initial healing has taken place, a week or so after surgery. They help to maintain and improve range, strength and coordination of muscle movements for speech and swallowing

➤ Advising on strategies to make speech clearer and swallowing easier and safer

➤ Ongoing review as the treatment and recovery progresses

Speech and language therapy takes place at the hospital where the treatment is given and sometimes locally after returning home. It may be required for anything from a few weeks to 12 to 18 months.

———•———

DIET AND NUTRITION

Aoife Gorham, Clinical Specialist Dietitian,
St James's Hospital, Dublin

Good nutrition involves eating enough of a wide variety of foods to make sure you get all the energy and nutrients you need. It can be difficult to eat enough before, during and after your treatment. The location of your tumour may make it more difficult to eat or drink. Sometimes side effects of treatment such as feeling sick, having a sore mouth or having problems swallowing can make it even harder to eat and cause unplanned weight loss.

Eating habits that are good for people with head and neck cancer can be very different from standard healthy-eating guidelines. When you have cancer you may need more nourishment from food, yet you may not feel like eating. If you are losing weight or struggling with your food, ask your doctor to refer you to a dietitian. Dietitians are trained in giving advice about diets that are safe, based on scientific evidence and that will help you to meet your nutritional needs.

If you have lost weight or are at risk of losing weight, your dietitian will recommend that you eat foods that are high in calories and protein. You may think this seems unhealthy but you should only need this diet for a short time while your appetite is poor. This will keep your body well nourished and help you to:

➤ Build up your strength and energy levels

➤ Keep up your weight. This can prevent radiotherapy treatment being delayed or rescheduled because your mask no longer fits properly

➤ Heal faster

➤ Keep well and avoid infections

➤ Feel better and be more active

➤ Manage the side effects of your illness and treatment better

➤ Reduce the need for nutrition-related hospital admissions/GP visits during your treatment

Tips on how to stay well nourished throughout your treatment if you have a poor appetite or are losing weight

➤ Eat foods high in protein and calories in the weeks before, during and after treatment, until your side effects have reduced and until your appetite has returned to normal

➤ Try to eat when your appetite is at its best. This may be breakfast time. Why not try a cooked breakfast or porridge and honey?

➤ A very full plate of food can put you off eating if you have a small appetite. Try having your food on a smaller plate to keep portions small. You can always go back for seconds if you still feel hungry

➤ If your appetite isn't good, eat small amounts regularly. Aim to eat five to six smaller meals throughout the day rather than the traditional three meals per day

➤ Don't skip meals and don't wait until you are hungry to eat. Try a few mouthfuls even if you are not hungry

➤ Drinking during meals may make you feel full, so sip only small amounts or, if you can, drink 30 minutes before or after your meal. If you are choosing a drink with your meal, choose a nourishing drink like full-fat milk. If your mouth is dry, you can add gravy or sauce to your food to help moisten it

➤ Choose full-fat versions of foods and drinks. Look for foods that are labelled 'thick and creamy' or 'luxury' and avoid diet or low-fat varieties

➤ Don't fill up on low-energy foods such as vegetables and fruit

➤ Try to make extra portions and freeze them or stock up on ready-made meals in advance for those days that you may not feel like or don't have the energy to cook

➤ Try adding extra energy and protein to your food and drinks by using some of the following:

  - *Full-fat milk*
  - *Skimmed milk powder*
  - *Double cream/sour cream/plain yoghurt*
  - *Peanut butter*
  - *Mayonnaise*
  - *Butter/margarine*
  - *Cream cheese*
  - *Hard cheese (can be grated and allowed to melt into food)*

Nourishing and supplementary drinks

Nourishing drinks like yoghurt drinks and milkshakes are an excellent source of both protein and energy and should be taken if you are losing weight or have a poor appetite. You should take your nourishing drinks between meals, not instead of meals. Your dietitian will advise you on how many nourishing drinks you need to have a day.

If you continue to have a poor appetite or are losing weight, your dietitian may recommend that you take some nutritional supplements to help boost the calories and protein in your diet. These nutritional supplements are available on prescription or over the counter in many different forms and flavours. Your dietitian will advise you on which is best for you and how many you need to take each day.

Side effects of radiotherapy and chemotherapy

Some patients may experience difficulties with eating because of their cancer before treatment starts and others may start to have problems during treatment.

The side effects of radiotherapy normally begin between the second and third weeks of treatment. These can get worse during the fourth and fifth week and last for about two to three weeks after treatment, though this can vary depending on your treatment plan. Your dietitian will be able to give you some helpful hints on coping with these side effects.

These are some of the side effects you may experience during and after your treatment:

- Dry mouth
- Sore mouth or throat
- Taste changes
- Feeling full quickly
- Nausea
- Vomiting
- Tiredness
- Diarrhoea
- Constipation

Different consistencies of diets and fluids

You may have been advised by your speech and language therapist to have a different texture or consistency of diet or fluids, e.g. soft diet, purée diet, minced and moist diet and/or thickened fluids. This is to allow you to swallow foods and fluids easily and safely. Your dietitian will advise you on how to ensure your diet is nutritionally balanced. If you have any questions or concerns about swallowing, please ask your doctor to refer you to the speech and language therapist.

Artificial nutrition support

Some patients may not be able to take enough food and fluids by mouth to meet their nutritional needs during their treatment, because of the location of their tumour or because of the side effects of their treatment. Some patients may need a feeding tube, which is a small plastic tube placed into your nose or stomach. Usually we can predict which patients may require these tubes and your doctor and dietitian will discuss this with you in detail before your treatment starts. Many patients have these tubes removed once they are able to take enough nourishment from diet and fluids alone to maintain their weight.

Complementary and alternative diets

In recent years complementary and alternative diets have become very popular, with much information available in books, on the internet and through the media. In some cases these diets can be harmful, difficult to follow and low in energy. You should treat any complementary or alternative diet with caution. If you are considering following one of these diets or are taking any nutritional supplements, please talk to your doctor or dietitian.

Please note this is general advice and does not replace any individualised advice you may have received from your dietitian or speech and language therapist.

———•———

TRACHEOSTOMY

Joy Norton, Post-graduate H.Dip ENT Nursing, Tracheostomy Safety Facilitator, St James's Hospital, Dublin

This section will help explain the function and role of a tracheostomy tube and why it is needed by some patients with head and neck cancers. I hope the information will answer some of your questions and reassure you about this part of your treatment.

What is a tracheostomy?

A tracheostomy is an opening that is made through the skin in the front of the neck into the trachea (windpipe). A tracheostomy tube is inserted into this opening to assist your breathing.

Why do I need one?

There are a number of reasons why a tracheostomy may be necessary. These include:

➤ After some operations to the mouth and neck area there can be swelling of your upper airway. The tracheostomy tube is inserted to bypass the swelling and ensure that air gets to your lungs. This tube is usually temporary and is removed once the swelling settles, approximately five to ten days after surgery

➤ Blockage of the windpipe due to tumour or swelling post-radiotherapy. This tracheostomy can be more long-term and you may need to be discharged with the tracheostomy tube in place

How does it work?

The tube is positioned in the centre of the neck. Instead of breathing air in and out through your nose and mouth, when a tracheostomy tube is in place, air will be directed in and out through the tube. Therefore, if you have a tracheostomy tube in place and oxygen is required, the mask is placed over the tube and not the face. You will breathe automatically through the tube and will not have to remind yourself to do so.

Will my speech be affected?

Initially, yes. When the tube is first inserted you will not be able to speak because breathing through the tracheostomy tube redirects air away from your vocal cords. This is temporary. If your voice box (larynx) is not affected by your condition, you should be able to speak using a Passy-Muir speaking valve and techniques you will be shown by the speech and language therapist.

Will I be able to eat?

A speech and language therapist will assess your swallow to ensure food and drink are not aspirated (i.e. do not go down the wrong way into the windpipe instead of the oesophagus). Once it is deemed safe you are usually allowed to eat and drink. You may find that certain foods and drinks are easier to swallow than others. Your dietitian and speech therapist will recommend a diet plan that will work best for you.

Sometimes after head and neck surgery you are not allowed to eat by mouth for a long time, so that your mouth can heal. A feeding tube may be inserted into your nose or into your tummy to enable you to receive the appropriate nutrition. It is very important that mouth/oral care is provided during this period.

OTHER PHYSICAL ISSUES

Humidification

Normally the air you breathe in is warmed and moistened as it passes through your nose and mouth on the way to your lungs. This process is called humidification. Humidification does not happen when air is inhaled through a tracheostomy tube. Therefore an external device needs to be used to add heat and moisture. There are a number of devices available. The tracheostomy safety facilitator or ward nurse will help you decide which is the most suitable for you.

Clearing secretions

While your tracheostomy tube is in place you may need help to clear secretions like sputum/phlegm that would normally be swallowed or coughed out. Suctioning is used for this purpose. This involves passing a small suction tube into your tracheostomy to manually suck out your secretions. It is performed by your nurse or physiotherapist, or you may be shown how to do it yourself.

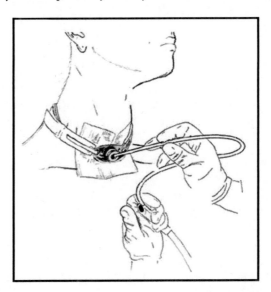

After surgery to the mouth or tongue you may find it difficult to swallow your own saliva and you may find that you have pooling secretions in your mouth. An oral Yankauer suction tip (a firm plastic suction tip with a bulbous head, which allows suction to take place without damaging surrounding structures) can be helpful to assist you in clearing these secretions. The nurse will ensure that your consultant is happy for you to use this as caution is warranted when using oral suction with new mouth grafts/flaps and extra care is needed not to damage them, so it will not be suitable for every patient.

Removal of your tracheostomy tube

If you had the tube inserted for surgery to the mouth and neck area, it is usually removed when all the swelling has subsided.

There are two different techniques used for its removal:

Technique 1

> Firstly, your tube will be downsized, i.e. changed to a smaller size

> The front opening will then be 'capped off' so that you get used to breathing through your nose and mouth again

> Once you can tolerate being 'capped off', and your doctor is happy with your overall condition, the tracheostomy tube is removed. This is not painful and you should not feel any discomfort

> An airtight dressing is applied over the exit site (where the tube was removed from). The exit site heals in approximately seven to ten days.

Technique 2

> The tracheostomy tube may be removed directly and downsizing and capping off unnecessary. The doctor will suture (stitch) the exit site immediately after the tube is removed; some local anaesthetic is injected around the site to make this as painless as possible. Sutures are removed after five days.

Looking after your tracheostomy at home (long-term tracheostomy)

Not all patients are suitable for decannulation (removal of the tube) and some will need to be prepared to be discharged with the tracheostomy tube in place. Before you leave hospital, both you and your family will be taught how to look after your tracheostomy at home. Also, your GP and local public health nurse will be available to support you at home.

When you go home with a tracheostomy tube in place, you will need one or more of the following pieces of equipment:

- ➤ Suction machine
- ➤ Suction catheters
- ➤ Nebuliser machine
- ➤ Room humidifier (Argos, approx €45)
- ➤ Shiley inner cannula green/clear
- ➤ Tube holders/ties
- ➤ Sofshield bib/Swedish nose (HME)

All, apart from the room humidifier, are ordered for you by the tracheostomy safety facilitator and are usually provided by your local health centre if you have a medical card. If you don't have a medical card the medical social worker will arrange one for you before you are discharged.

Living with a tracheostomy tube

Having a tracheostomy tube does not mean that you can't live a very full and active life. The following are some tips to help you to remain as active and healthy as possible while your tube is in place.

Appearance

As a tracheostomy tube can be seen on the front of your neck, it does alter your appearance. It may take some time to get used to your neck looking different. Some people find it helpful to wear a scarf or a cravat. There are also mock polo-neck T-shirts available from your speech therapist. It will help if you talk to your friends, relatives and your nurses about how you feel about your appearance, so that they can give you the support you need.

Importance of humidification

When you are going out make sure your tracheostomy is covered with humidifier bibs or a Swedish nose. Be careful around animals, because of stray hairs, and around open fires, because of the ash. If ash or pet hair are inhaled your airway will become irritated, causing respiratory distress (difficulty breathing).

Another way of ensuring the sputum doesn't get too thick and dry is to make sure you keep yourself hydrated. Ensure you have plenty of fluids, either by mouth or PEG tube.

Bathing and showering

➤ When you shower, use one of the blue plastic shower bibs over the Sofshield bib or Swedish nose. These will be provided by the hospital or your local health centre. They tie around the neck and are secured with Velcro. If water gets into your tracheostomy tube, it will make you cough a lot, as it goes into the lungs.

➤ It is safe to have a bath provided there is no water contact with your tracheostomy tube.

➤ Swimming should be avoided and is only possible with the use of specialised equipment and instruction.

Work

A tracheostomy tube will not prevent you from doing most jobs. Talk to your doctor or nurse if your work involves a lot of dust (e.g. farming or carpentry), or heavy lifting, or if you have any questions about your work.

Sport

Many sports can be continued with a tracheostomy tube in place. However contact sports like boxing, rugby or Gaelic football are not advised. Again, talk to your doctor or nurse and they will be happy to advise you.

Overall health

Good quality of life with a tracheostomy is not just about looking after your tube. It involves all the other elements that make up a healthy lifestyle. Eating well, getting enough sleep, taking exercise, getting out and about and continuing to do the fun things that you enjoy are all important. Sexual activity can also be continued. It is important also that you talk to and include your family, friends and health professionals during this time, so that they can give you the support that you need.

Should you feel as if you are getting a cold, contact your GP for a check-up, as it is not advisable that you wait for it to improve.

Follow-up care

The entire tube needs to be changed in clinic every month. You will be given an appointment on discharge. The tube change will be carried out by the tracheostomy safety facilitator or an ENT doctor.

PSYCHO-ONCOLOGY

Allison Connolly, Counselling Psychologist, Psycho-Oncology Department, St Luke's Hospital, Dublin

For many the diagnosis of head and neck cancer comes so swiftly there is little time to prepare, and treatment may start almost immediately, leaving you little time to process the news. Indeed, your diagnosis may be the first time you have heard of head and neck cancer. As you adjust to the news, there can be a sense that the diagnosis demarcates your life into life before cancer and life after cancer. But this is not always the case; for some, the cancer journey becomes part of their life story rather than a defining landmark of change. For each person diagnosed with head and neck cancer, the cancer journey will have unique aspects, but there are often overlapping themes.

Ultimately there is no singular way to cope, but there is a broad sketch of what is known to buffer low mood in times of stress, change and uncertainty, which is undoubtedly brought on when undergoing treatment for head and neck cancer. While information on coping well is widely available through cancer support agencies, some people do choose to meet with a psychologist for one-to-one help. The reasons a person with head and neck cancer will choose to meet with a psychologist vary. For some, life stressors prior to the diagnosis of cancer contribute to a sea of emotional upheaval and add to the challenge of adjusting to the illness and its treatment. Others need more pragmatic input around sleep and management of fatigue and pain. Changes in body image, ability to communicate, the stress of disfigurement, perceived stigma and the resulting impact on confidence levels are often dealt with during psychological therapy in this context. However, not every patient will choose to meet with a psychologist during the course of their cancer journey and often the support of family and close friends will allow for these issues to be digested independently.

Challenges and concerns during treatment

Good coping will be influenced by the physical and emotional demands that each person faces, both in their daily life and in their medical treatment. Broadly speaking, stress levels are at their highest at the point of confirmed diagnosis and generally recede during treatment. This anxiety is a natural response to feeling heightened levels of unease in a new situation. In addition, anxiety will rise and fall in response to the challenges associated with different stages of the disease and treatment.

Responses can be variable, and may even be contradictory. Initially, you may feel numb to the news of diagnosis, followed by feelings of anxiety in the lead up to your first radiotherapy session. Your feelings may level out again over the course of radiotherapy treatment. Some feel shock in every fibre of their being, followed by a keen need to keep anxiety at bay by gathering information and taking a matter-of-fact approach. Anxiety can also take a more exaggerated form with radiotherapy treatment/mask fitting during planning but can often be attended to by learning tricks and tips for managing these feelings by meeting with a psychologist in advance of mask fitting. If you have a history of claustrophobia or are worried about feeling claustrophobic, let your medical team know in advance of mask fitting, so they can support you and address your concerns.

Inwardly, fears and self-questioning are a normal part of the process of coming to terms with head and neck cancer. It can take tremendous courage to continue to engage in the aspects of life and the activities that are meaningful and valuable to you. Maintaining a sense of involvement in your life is most effective in aiding adjustment if undertaken at the point of diagnosis and continued beyond the completion of treatment.

Difficulties with eating can be a central challenge. Head and neck cancer has a unique impact among cancer types in its impact on shared experiences we often take for granted, such as sharing a meal and being cared for with food. Strong feelings can be associated with this aspect of the disease for both the person with cancer and their family members. The demands these difficulties place on time, thought and energy are enormous and often poignantly felt. It cannot be overestimated how daily life is affected, as food represents not only a way to sustain life but also a vehicle for interaction and socialising with others.

Physical changes can bring feelings of shame, discomfort and changes in social life. They raise tricky decisions around managing celebrations such as weddings, birthdays and holidays. Often you must reconcile yourself to what you can no longer eat, which may involve a process of trial and error. Partners or carers may need to work hard to keep motivation levels up to maintain good nutrition. Cravings or fantasies about food and eating may form a part of the experience, as a 'new normal' develops.

Coping strategies

➤ Know your needs. Follow your own lead

➤ Don't feel you need to be any particular way (e.g. sometimes people feel pressure to be positive)

➤ Think over whether you are someone who likes a lot of information or whether you prefer less. Let your medical team and others around you know so they can tailor the information they give you

➤ Consider which people you wish to have around and who you find difficult to be with

➤ At times it may be necessary to take a pragmatic outlook and a determined stance to 'get through it'. At other times it may be helpful to be patient and kind with yourself

➤ Feelings are temporary and transient. Use tools that help to keep perspective, whether it's time out alone, a comforting visit with an understanding friend (who won't put pressure on you to talk if this isn't physically possible at the time), or any activity that brings comfort in times of distress or hardship

➤ Establish goals, which may be immediate and concrete. It's important to have the feeling you are doing something that matters, whether it is looking after your diet and your skin (areas of redness, or scarring), or planning small rewards to keep you going when morale is low

➤ Pacing yourself is an enormous challenge but it is important in maintaining a sense of well-being and in offsetting fatigue. Pacing can require lots of time and reflection to get the balance right, and involves knowing your body, using short activity periods, scheduled rest, routines, prioritising and switching tasks

Challenges and concerns following treatment

All the changes the disease causes are brought to the foreground in the aftermath of treatment. The greatest expenditure of energy may not lie in the day-to-day maintenance and care of the site of cancer and oral or wound care after surgery, but rather in the significant thoughts, feelings and worries attached to fears of recurrence, or the process of re-establishing a sense of physical safety after diagnosis and treatment, when many aspects of one's physical body may be temporarily or permanently altered. In fact, the physical aspects of worry (chest pain, poor sleep) can often heighten our perception that our body is still in danger, even after treatment. Once treatment is finished it is common to feel somewhat abandoned by the sudden absence of daily medical care, and there can be a sense of waiting in suspense until the follow-up scans. Fears around treatment and recurrence can be counterbalanced by information from your medical team and regular follow-ups with them.

It is common to wonder where your levels of anxiety rest in the spectrum. Problematic anxiety will feel persistent, disruptive to daily life and overwhelming.

When low mood strikes, emotions tend to shape our thinking. At times your confidence in yourself may suffer (e.g. 'I'm no good.') or your view of the future may be affected ('Things will never change.')

Undoubtedly the biggest challenge of going through cancer lies in our capacity to be hard on ourselves and to search for answers in the form of undeserved self-blame. During the worst spells, your view of the world may seem darkened ('Everyone thinks I'm different now'). Feelings can include sadness, guilt and anxiety. In times of self-doubt social situations can be very uncomfortable, particularly in one's community and out of concern for the reactions of others. It is easy to underestimate the power of looking at yourself in the mirror, self-care, grooming and maintaining an interactive link with family and friends as part of the process of adaptation.

Your physical changes may also affect how others react to you. Not everyone knows how to react to people who have had cancer or who have changed physically due to cancer or treatment. Your relationship to your body may vary depending on where you are (e.g. St Luke's Hospital versus your local shop). Planning quick and prepared answers, regarding the illness, its treatment and the visible changes, that you are comfortable sharing (e.g. one response with less detail for the shopkeeper you see regularly, another response that would be suitable for an acquaintance etc.) will help maintain a sense of control and choice when you are dealing with discomfort in social situations.

Coping strategies

The biggest challenge is getting the right balance between the need for autonomy and the need for connection. Both autonomy and closeness are natural human needs.

> ➤ Find a way to say 'I need time out for me.' Allow others time for the news and the changes to sink in

> ➤ Give others who matter in your life the facts, and if you think it will be helpful, get them involved

> ➤ Looking back on other challenging moments in your life may provide a roadmap of what is helpful and of what gets you through difficult times. Equally, new coping skills may need to be developed

Finding your footing

Coping is often not a stable or set in stone route. It is particularly important to acknowledge and leave space in your life for concerns about cancer recurrence to be heightened during the periods before review appointments with your medical team. Allowing for ups and downs is a challenging but vital skill.

Calming techniques, including the use and practice of deep breathing, progressive muscular relaxation using guided CDs, online resources or smartphone apps, and meditation/mindfulness are all scientifically proven ways to ease anxiety and relax the body. Low-lying stress and tension can be cumulative and they can have an impact on sleep and appetite. While some prefer to practise relaxation in private, many find attending formal classes in community centres to be invaluable as a way to build a new skill that will be useful during future stressful experiences. Regardless of your approach, the most important aspect of recovery is finding a pace and an approach that works for you.

DENTAL AND ORAL HEALTH

Wenda Thomas, RDH, Staff Dental Hygienist,
Dublin Dental University Hospital

Sarah Troute, RDH, Staff Dental Hygienist,
Dublin Dental University Hospital

Denise MacCarthy, Senior Lecturer Consultant in Restorative Dentistry
and Periodontology, School of Dental Science, Trinity College Dublin

A dental assessment before radiation treatment, and ideally before surgery and chemotherapy, is part of established best practice for patient care. This is because radiotherapy affects the salivary glands, resulting in a dry mouth due to lack of saliva. Saliva contains enzymes that help digest food. It also contains antibodies that help protect against infections of the mouth and throat.

The jawbone is also affected by radiation treatment, which may result in severe infection and non-healing after trauma such as a dental extraction. This is called osteoradionecrosis (ORN).

The severity of dry mouth is unpredictable, but with the use of Intensity-modulated radiation therapy (IMRT) dryness may be reduced. Dry mouth following radiotherapy often results in dietary changes, which may lead to dental decay.

Guidelines for keeping your mouth and teeth healthy

> ➤ Brush and floss at least once daily

➤ Avoid sugary foods and drinks. Read labels on packaging to find hidden sugars

➤ Do not smoke, and if you drink alcohol, do so moderately

➤ Visit your dentist and dental hygienist regularly for routine care

➤ Keep your mouth moist and lubricated

Before radiation treatment

➤ Teeth in poor condition will be extracted

➤ Teeth in the high-radiation dose area will be assessed carefully because if these teeth are in poor condition or are very close to the tumour, they may need to be extracted at this point as it is much more difficult and risky to do so after radiation treatment

➤ A plan for your oral health will be developed, including advice on oral hygiene and diet

➤ You will be given jaw exercises to maintain jaw movement. It is vital that mouth opening is maintained as much as possible, as surgery and radiation can cause a reduction. If you or the dentist cannot reach your teeth in the future, problems cannot be treated

➤ A radiation stent may be requested by the radiation oncologist. This is a plastic device to hold the jaws apart and move tissue (e.g. the tongue) out of the radiation field. This helps to spare healthy tissue from the effects of radiation. The stent may also have lead lining to shield tissue from radiation

➤ Your teeth will be cleaned and scaled

Preventing dental decay and extractions

When there is a reduction in your saliva flow (dry mouth), you are at increased risk of developing decay in your teeth. Dental decay is caused by acid demineralisation of the tooth. The acid is the by-product of the action of bacteria in dental plaque on food, especially sugar.

Fluoride is scientifically proven to remineralise teeth affected by decay. In Ireland, fluoride is generally available in our tap water and also in fluoridated toothpaste. When you are at a high risk of decay more concentrated fluoride application is advisable.

Chlorhexidine gel will control bacteria in dental plaque that forms on your teeth. You must limit the sugar in your diet and apply topical fluoride and chlorhexidine gels/pastes to your teeth. This can be done either by applying the gel with a toothbrush or by wearing specially made medication trays that fit over your teeth like a mouthguard. Daily application will help to replace the effects of the saliva. Gel applications should be continued long-term, and it is important to continue to use the fluoride/chlorhexidine even if you have a PEG tube. Your dentist will check your saliva flow and dental decay at six months and one year.

Healthy gums and healthy teeth

Periodontal disease includes gingivitis (bleeding gums) and periodontitis (destruction of the bone that holds the teeth in place). It is caused by the build-up of bacterial dental plaque, a soft colourless film of bacteria that forms on the tooth surface soon after brushing. Your immune response to the plaque bacteria also has a role in the severity of periodontitis. Successful treatment is dependent on effective brushing and cleaning in between your teeth.

The following sequence of treatment is generally used to treat gum disease:

➤ Oral hygiene instruction and plaque control – brushing and cleaning in between the teeth

➤ You will be encouraged to quit smoking

➤ Your dentist or dental hygienist will scale and polish the surfaces of your teeth i.e. remove the plaque and calculus (tartar)

➤ If the destruction of the supporting bone is too severe, extraction may be best

➤ Regular follow-up and care is essential in the long term management of the condition

Dry mouth

Dry mouth is a side effect of radiation treatment on the saliva-producing glands. The dryness may be a result of reduction or a total absence of saliva. It usually starts during or immediately following radiation treatment. Depending on the level of injury to the saliva glands some of your saliva flow may return over the following year. If you have no remaining saliva gland function and are totally dry, there are a number of saliva substitutes on the market. Ask your dentist or nurse to recommend one. You may have to try a few before you find one that suits. Dry mouth makes eating, opening your mouth, speaking, swallowing and sleeping difficult.

Tips for managing dry mouth

- ➤ Take good care of your mouth and keep it clean. Saliva acts as a natural mouthwash so you need to make up for this loss of natural protection

- ➤ Do not smoke, and if you drink alcohol, do so in moderation

- ➤ Avoid frequent sugar in your diet. Use fluoride and chlorhexidine gel as recommended by your dentist

- ➤ Moisturise your lips with lip balm or water-soluble moisturiser

- ➤ Carry a small bottle of still water to sip during the day and keep water beside your bed

- ➤ Put a humidifier beside your bed

- ➤ Chew sugar-free chewing gum. This may help to stimulate saliva flow if there is some remaining saliva gland function. There are also some tablets your doctor can prescribe to help stimulate saliva

- ➤ Currently available saliva substitutes include BioXtra, Biotene, Oralieve, Saliva Orthana and Mouth Kote. If you have your own natural teeth, avoid products that contain citric acid, as these will erode your teeth. Always read the list of ingredients

- ➤ Try flavourless salad oil at night to lubricate your mouth

- ➤ Increase your intake of fluids. Avoid too much fruit juice, as it is acidic and will make your teeth sensitive. Tap water is best

- ➤ At meal times, eat soft creamy foods; use gravy and sauces and drink water when you are eating

- ➤ You should avoid very hot or spicy foods, hard, coarse food (e.g. crackers and toast), smoking, alcohol, lemon glycerine swabs

Mouth opening

Following surgery or radiotherapy to the mouth, head and neck, you may experience a reduced mouth opening. This makes daily oral hygiene and professional dental care very difficult. You will be advised about the three finger test, which uses your fingers to measure your mouth opening. If you notice that your mouth opening is becoming a problem, you may be advised to use a mechanical device to help. One such device is the TheraBite. You should ask your dentist or speech therapist about this if you think it might help you.

Maxillofacial prosthodontics and rehabilitation following surgery

If you have cancer that requires surgery on the jawbone, part of your jaws may be removed to treat the cancer. Following a period of healing, tissue that has been removed will often need to be replaced. This may be done with a denture, an obturator or with the aid of dental implants. An obturator is a prosthetic device used to restore function in acquired defects of the palate that are the result of the surgical treatment of cancer. These defects predispose the patient to hypernasal speech, fluid leakage into the nasal cavity, and difficulty speaking. Bone and soft tissue loss in the mandible (lower jaw) are more difficult to replace and may need the use of dental implants. These are titanium metal inserts placed in the jaw to help retain prosthetic appliances. Implants are also used to retain ear, eye and nose prostheses.

Dental and oral care of the mouth, head and neck cancer patient is a very specialised area and is provided in dedicated units. Routine dental care such as fillings, root canal treatments, crowns and scaling can be carried out by the general dentist. However, the risk of ORN is permanent and dental extractions from irradiated bone should always be done in a specialised unit.

With excellent oral care at home, including oral hygiene and use of decay prevention gels, it should be possible to retain your teeth. Having your own natural teeth is a great benefit following cancer treatment, especially if you have a dry mouth.

ORAL HYGIENE, TOOTH DECAY CONTROL AND DRY MOUTH PRODUCTS

Listed here are products that are mentioned in the memoirs. These are products that patients have found helpful. You may or may not find that they work for you but they are worth trying. Always read the list of ingredients.

➤ Try various products for dry mouth; personal preference is important

➤ Avoid products containing alcohol

➤ Avoid products containing citric acid if you have your own natural teeth, as the acid may erode your teeth

➤ Use sugar-free chewing gum

NAME	ACTIVE INGREDIENT	USE
Corsodyl gel Periokin gel	Chlorhexidine digluconate 1%	Antiseptic gel for **infection prevention**
Corsodyl mouthwash Periokin mouthwash	0.2% OR 0.1% Chlorhexidine gluconate Periokin is alcohol free	Mouthwash for **infection prevention**
Corsodyl daily mouthwash	0.06% Chlorhexidine, 250ppm sodium fluoride, alcohol free	Mouthwash for **infection prevention**
Corsodyl Daily Gum & Tooth Paste	Sodium bicarbonate	For **cleaning teeth**
Listerine	Thymol, eucalyptol, alcohol	Mouthwash for **infection prevention**
Listerine Zero	Alcohol free, thymol, eucalyptol	Mouthwash for **infection prevention**
BioXtra gel Biothene gel Oralieve gel	Lactoperoxidase, lysozyme, lactoferrin, glucose oxidase, calcium lactate, potassium thiocyanate	Gel to lubricate **dry mouth**
BioXtra mouthwash Biotene mouthwash Oralieve mouthwash	Lactoperoxidase, lysozyme, lactoferrin, glucose oxidase, calcium lactate, potassium thiocyanate	Mouthwash to lubricate **dry mouth**
Stoppers 4 Dry Mouth (only available in USA)	Lactoperoxidase, lysozyme, lactoferrin, glucose oxidase calcium lactate, potassium thiocyanate	Spray to lubricate **dry mouth**
A.S. Saliva Orthana	Contains porcine derived gastric mucin.	Rinse/spray to lubricate **dry mouth**

Mouth Kote	Eriodictyon crassifolium (yerba santa)	Spray to lubricate **dry mouth**
Glandosane	Carboxymethylcellulose, minerals (Na, K, CaCl), lemon	Spray to lubricate **dry mouth**
GC Dry Mouth Gel (only available from dentist)	Cellulose gum, carrageenan, sodium citrate	Gel to lubricate **dry mouth**
Elizabeth Arden Eight Hour Cream Skin Protectant		Moisturises lips
Colgate Duraphat Daily Mouthwash	500ppm sodium fluoride, alcohol free	Mouthwash to **control dental decay**
Sensodyne Gentle Mouthwash	250ppm fluoride, potassium chloride, cetyl pyrimidine chloride, alcohol free	Mouthwash to **control decay** and **sensitive teeth**
Colgate Duraphat Toothpaste	2800 or 5000ppm sodium fluoride	Toothpaste to **control dental decay**
Colgate FlouriGard Daily Mouth Rinse	Sodium fluoride 225ppm	Mouthwash to **control dental decay**
GC Tooth Mousse and GC Tooth Mousse Plus (only available from dentist)	Regular: calcium, phosphate Plus: calcium, phosphate, fluoride	Cream to **control tooth decay**

———•———

PHYSIOTHERAPY

Joanne Dowds, Respiratory Clinical Specialist,
St James's Hospital, Dublin

Jean-Marc Monseux, Lymphoedema Physiotherapist,
St James's Hospital, Dublin

The focus of any physiotherapist is to return whatever function the client has lost through injury, surgery or the effects of surgery. In the case of those with head, neck and mouth cancer, physiotherapy has a more specific role in reducing pain and swelling, clearing secretions, improving movement of the head, neck and shoulders and returning maximum function to the arms.

We generally teach those who have undergone surgery for head, neck and mouth cancer how to clear their own chest secretions. This is usually through breathing exercises, by teaching the patient how to cough most effectively.

Occasionally we may need to use other techniques like suctioning to help remove secretions. Suctioning is where we use a small tube to suck out any phlegm, either from the mouth, the back of the throat or, if the patient has a tracheostomy, we can suction through that. Suctioning is not something any healthcare professional does lightly. We try to only do suction when we feel we have to, as it can be uncomfortable for the patient.

Our other big role after surgery is moving the patient out of bed for the first time. This can be a very nerve-wracking experience, particularly when the patient is in an intensive care environment. Sitting up and getting out of bed is a big event and a worthwhile one. The most important aspect is to reassure the patient and make sure she or he knows how we are going to move. We break down the smooth movement of lying to sitting into a series of smaller, more gentle moves. The patient needs to be talked through all of it and generally this is where the therapist's bossy tone of voice comes to the fore. One of the biggest things to make the patient aware of is the unusual sensation of having a heavy head; this is only due to the surgery and improves quickly, but it isn't usually until that first unsupported sit-up that the patient complains of being unable to support their own head. So occasionally I support someone's head while they get out of bed and hope that their body comes along with me!

Once the immediate effects of the surgery (wound pain, groggy feeling, fatigue) begin to ease, the role of the physiotherapist becomes about getting people back to their normal levels of exercise, whatever that may be. We try to talk to each patient about what activities they were able to do before surgery and what they would like to be able to continue to do afterwards.

A common problem in the months following surgery is pain and stiffness in the shoulders and neck. This can have implications for work, driving and even general activities like washing your hair, getting dressed or carrying bags of shopping. Activities such as swimming and Pilates yoga can be helpful activities for these issues. Physiotherapy can help too; we can give advice about how best to regain strength and movement and then help to deal with any shortened muscles, tight scars, swelling or stiff joints. These are not quick fixes; it does take time. It can be a long journey back, and I hope that physiotherapists can be good travelling companions to the head, neck and mouth cancer survivor on their journey.

———◆———

COMPLEMENTARY THERAPIES

Yoga

Anne L'Hénoret, Yoga Teacher and Holistic Therapist (ITEC)

The yoga techniques I used in my recovery from tongue cancer were extremely simple and can be used by any patient regardless of age or level of fitness. There is no need for prior experience to benefit. I also encourage you to persevere with the tasks you are given by speech therapists and physiotherapists.

Little and often is the way to go, especially if you are working through fatigue or pain. When you stretch, go to the edge of your pain threshold and to the edge of the muscular tightness, then stay there and breathe. Be gentle yet determined. Always breathe through any effort, and the feeling it brings up. Don't hold your breath if you get sore or upset. Breathing through pain and upset doesn't just help with physical mobility and strength, it also allows you to become more familiar with, and to accept, your changed body or face.

Ask your medical team how soon you can start stretching and massaging the affected areas. Once the wounds are closed and you get the go ahead, don't wait. Muscles and body tissue stiffen fast, but they also loosen fast, so do a little often, as soon as you are allowed.

Yoga exercises for mobility and strength

> ➤ You need to maintain wide mouth opening to eat comfortably and to receive dental care in the future. Stretch the jaw open several times a day. For a change you can also slide the lower jaw side to-side or draw circles with it.

➤ If your neck becomes stiff from the surgery itself, or from the stress, effective stretches include: tilting the head from side to side; turning the head on a horizontal plane as if looking behind you; moving the head forward and back. Do a few movements without holding first, to loosen up, then hold each stretch for a number of breaths to really increase mobility. Also practise turning the head on a horizontal plane to look back, then look up and down slightly in that position.

➤ If you have had a neck dissection and your shoulder is affected, it may tilt forward. This can cause weakness and pain in the shoulder and arm and can even affect the tone of the breast. Follow your physiotherapist's advice initially, and then combine and maintain it with yoga or Pilates posture exercises. You need to actively strengthen the back and shoulder muscles that pull the shoulder-blade back, to compensate for the tendency of the front shoulder to fall forward. A simple exercise that you can do sitting down is to pretend you are using a bow and arrow. Start with your arms straight in front of you, fists touching. Bend the elbow of the affected side and pull it back as you twist around to the same side. Don't hike the shoulder towards the ear, and reach your other arm straight in front of you. Look up the yoga postures called *locust* and *cobra* and practise the variations where your hands are neither touching the floor nor clasped behind your back, so as to make your shoulders work more. The *dog* pose practised on the elbows and forearms is really excellent for recovering shoulder positioning.

➤ Strengthening the muscles at the front of the neck and throat helps to recover your swallow, compensate for a weak front shoulder and circulate the lymph in the neck. A simple exercise is to lie flat on your back and lift your head to look at your toes.

Radiotherapy causes rigidity in the tissues, so whether it is the tongue, the jaw or the neck, stretching the affected area increases mobility and helps it to feel more like before. Use the stretches above and those given to you by the team.

Always keep the eyes, the jaw, the face muscles, the hands, the whole body relaxed. Breathe. Yoga breathing is two things:

1. Being aware of your breath while being mindful of how you feel

2. Using your breath as a tool for relaxation and focus

Yoga for anxiety

Feelings of anxiety are a normal part of the experience of cancer. They may be mild and manageable, or they may overwhelm you to the point of panic. This can happen in the waiting room before hearing test results, or in the middle of the night when you can't talk to anyone. It may happen before going under anaesthetic for an operation or before having an injection. It may even happen after the end of treatment. Your breath can become shallow and your chest can feel tight; if it is severe you could get dizzy and feel you cannot breathe. Your body is going into panic mode but you always have the tool to stop it. Simply make each breath long and slow. Inhale for a count of ten and exhale for a count of ten until you are calm.

Yoga for pain management

Working with breath and mindfulness is great for pain management. This simple tool is always at your disposal. Use your breath and also notice your attitude. Be aware that most of our suffering comes not from the physical or practical problems we encounter, but from how we choose to respond to them. This is true on an emotional level if we try to fight something we cannot avoid, but it is also true on a physical level: we often tighten additional muscles when we feel pain or stress. This creates even more stress. If you feel pain, first relax the whole of your body, breathe mindfully and slowly, visualise the 'in breath' going into the painful area, bringing it well-being, and on the 'out breath' visualise the pain leaving the area, and feel the body relaxing even more.

Yoga for stressful situations

Mouth cancer treatment and side effects involve unpleasant and threatening experiences such as choking on food or drink, having cameras and feeding tubes inserted into your nose or mouth, tracheostomy with its associated problems and feelings of claustrophobia under the radiotherapy mask. These situations are stressful as your body may feel its survival is endangered. By staying calm you get through the unpleasantness and your mind can stay rational and do what is required. Use your nose to breathe if your throat is blocked. Keep your breathing slow and even. Inhale and exhale for the same count.

You may find using an affirmation is helpful. For example, during my radiotherapy sessions, I would settle into stillness under the mask, and as I breathed mindfully I would say in my head, 'Breathe in the benefits, breathe out the side effects.' This helped me to stay still and to come to terms with the fact that I was willingly doing something to my body that was both healing and harmful. Come up with one that works for you.

Massage

Lymphatic drainage massage is very useful for reducing swelling around scar tissue. This is healthy and also improves appearance. For example, after a neck dissection there can be swelling in the neck above the scar. Lymph massage is very, very light – a feather's touch almost. Use the flat of the fingers to gently move the superficial layers of skin in little semicircles away from the scar. This moves stagnating lymph to be reintegrated into the main lymphatic circulation.

For the muscles and body tissue that feel stiff from treatment, a stronger massage is required. This is about getting fresh blood and nutrients into the tissues and getting toxins out. For this you can use a larger area of the fingers and palm and apply firmer movements that reach the deeper layers of tissues. When the scar is well healed, don't be afraid to massage the scar itself and the surrounding area.

Dermatix is an excellent silicone-based product that reduces redness and lumpiness of scar tissue. It can usually be used about six weeks after surgery but check with your medical team before you use it. It also improves older scar tissue. Whether you are massaging Dermatix into the scar, or massaging moisturiser into dry skin after radiotherapy, or just doing your everyday grooming, a couple of minutes of massage promotes good circulation, suppleness and comfort in the area.

NB: THE FOLLOWING INFORMATION ABOUT COMPLEMENTARY THERAPIES WAS SOURCED ON THE INTERNET

Reiki (www.reiki.ie)

Reiki is a Japanese technique for stress reduction and relaxation that also promotes healing. It is administered by 'laying on hands' and is based on the idea that an invisible life-force energy flows through us and is what causes us to be alive. If our life-force energy is low, we are more likely to get sick or to feel stress; if it is high, we are more capable of being happy and healthy. The word reiki is made of two Japanese words: *rei,* which means 'God's wisdom' or 'the higher power', and *ki,* which means 'life-force energy'. So reiki is actually 'spiritually guided life-force energy'. Reiki treats the whole person, including body, emotions, mind and spirit, aiming to create beneficial effects such as relaxation and feelings of peace, security and well-being.

Acupuncture (www.mayoclinic.com)

Acupuncture is a complementary medical practice that involves stimulating certain points on the body, most often with a needle penetrating the skin, to alleviate pain or to treat various diseases. Developed in China, numerous recent studies conducted by scientists in Europe and the United States have found that acupuncture is at least moderately effective in treating pain and nausea.

Tai chi (www.mayoclinic.com)

Tai chi is an ancient Chinese tradition that today is practised as a graceful form of exercise. It involves a series of movements performed in a slow, focused manner and accompanied by deep breathing. Tai chi, also called tai chi chuan, is a non-competitive, self-paced system of gentle physical exercise and stretching. Each posture flows into the next without pause, ensuring that your body is in constant motion. Tai chi has many different styles. Each style may have its own subtle emphasis on various tai chi principles and methods. There are also variations within each style. Some may focus on health maintenance, while others focus on the martial arts aspect of tai chi. Tai chi is low impact and puts minimal stress on muscles and joints, making it generally safe for all ages and fitness levels. In fact, because tai chi is low impact, it may be especially suitable if you're an older adult who otherwise may not exercise. You may also find tai chi appealing because it's inexpensive, requires no special equipment and can be done indoors or out, either alone or in a group.

Pilates (www.mayoclinic.com)

Pilates is a method of exercise that consists of low-impact flexibility and muscular strength and endurance movements. Pilates emphasises use of the abdominals, lower back, hips and thighs.

———◆———

MANAGING THE FINANCIAL IMPACT OF CANCER

Tony Carlin, Head Medical Social Worker, St Luke's Hospital, Dublin

A cancer diagnosis frequently brings with it the added burden of financial worries. Therefore it is helpful to have a basic knowledge of the various benefits and entitlements for which you may qualify. Advice and helpful hints on how to navigate your way through the application processes for various social welfare benefits, allowances and the medical card can help to significantly minimise the stress. The following will provide some assistance in this regard.

Citizens Information

A most useful service of which you should be aware at the outset is Citizens

Information, which provides a comprehensive frequently updated repository of information about benefits, entitlements, medical cards, legal and employment rights etc. Its website is www.citizensinformation.ie. The service is also contactable at lo-call 1890 777121, Monday to Friday, 9.00 a.m. to 9.00 p.m. and at 260 drop-in locations nationwide.

Social welfare payments

The welfare payments you are most likely to be eligible for when you have cancer are Illness Benefit, Invalidity Pension or Disability Allowance. Illness Benefit is aimed at people whose illness is likely to be short-term. To qualify you have to have made a sufficient number of PRSI contributions prior to becoming unwell. You are also required to send in certificates signed by your GP to the Department of Social Protection on a weekly basis. This benefit can last for up to two years. However, in the event that you will be unable to return to work in the long-term due to your illness and you have been claiming Illness Benefit for at least 12 months, you may then qualify for an Invalidity Pension. This is again based on your PRSI contributions. If you have not made the necessary number of contributions, you can apply for a Disability Allowance. This is means assessed and requires you to be also medically assessed either by your GP or a consultant. If you are on an Invalidity Pension or Disability Allowance you may also qualify for a free travel pass and extra benefits such as an electricity or gas allowance, a telephone allowance and a free television licence.

The Partial Capacity Benefit is a relatively new scheme, which allows you to return to employment if you have a reduced capacity to work, and to continue to receive a payment from the Department of Social Protection. To qualify for this you need to have been receiving Illness Benefit for at least six months or be on an Invalidity Pension.

If you are caring for a person with cancer you may qualify for Carer's Benefit or Carer's Allowance. The former is based on contributions while the latter is means assessed. If you are on a Carer's Allowance you may also be eligible for the extra benefits referred to above and an annual respite care grant. If you are already on a social welfare payment, you may be still eligible for a half Carer's Allowance while retaining your other payment. If you are caring for an incapacitated person and are in employment, you are entitled by law to 104 weeks of unpaid carer's leave while at the same time preserving all your employment rights. For more information, you should contact the Employment Rights Information Unit, at lo-call 1890 201615.

With the exception of the application forms and certificates for Illness Benefit which are provided by the GP, all other application forms and information booklets for the above benefits and allowances can be downloaded from the Department of Social Protection's website (www.welfare.ie) or picked up from your local social welfare office. The main number for the Department of Social Protection is (01) 7043000 or lo-call 1890 928400.

If your application for any social welfare payment is refused, you can appeal this decision, but you need to do so within a short period.

Supplementary Welfare Allowance

If you have cancer and do not qualify for any of the above payments, you may be eligible for Supplementary Welfare Allowance. Also, if you have claimed for a social welfare benefit, allowance or pension, which has not yet come through, and you have no other means of income, you may qualify for this allowance. This payment helps to tide people over during emergencies and difficult times. You may also get help with special needs like rent or mortgage interest payments or for urgent or exceptional needs. The payment is a basic weekly allowance and is means tested. It is administered by community welfare officers who were previously employed by the HSE. However, since 2011 they have been employed by the Department of Social Protection. They are based either in health centres or in social welfare offices and are occasionally referred to as 'relieving officers'. As above, if you are refused a payment, you can appeal the decision.

Medical cards

There is a popular misconception that if you have a cancer diagnosis you are automatically entitled to a medical card. This is not the case. Eligibility for a medical card is based solely on means. There is, however, an emergency card process in place where a medical card can be provided in 24 hours on request if you meet one of the following criteria:

> ➤ You are in palliative care and terminally ill

> ➤ You are homeless and in need of urgent medical care

> ➤ You have a serious medical condition that requires urgent medical care

> ➤ You are a child in foster care or an asylum seeker in need of urgent medical care

All medical cards are now processed in a central office in Finglas in Dublin and if all information required for the application is submitted in the first instance, the processing time is usually 10 to 15 days. You can check the status of your application by logging on to www.medicalcard.ie and quoting your reference number, which you will be given after you make your application. You can also make direct contact with the office on (01) 8647100 or lo-call 1890 252919.

If you have a medical card and live in the HSE Eastern or North Eastern region, you are covered for treatment in the Dental Hospital.

Helpful hints for form filling and following up applications

When filling out application forms for social welfare and medical cards there are a number of useful tips, which may help to make the process less stressful and save a lot of valuable time.

- ➤ Always use black pen and write clearly
- ➤ Get help if necessary
- ➤ Do not leave boxes or sections free. Instead, cross out, or write N/A (not applicable)
- ➤ Make sure you have signed the form in all the appropriate places
- ➤ Have someone check the form before you send it
- ➤ If you can, get a letter from your social worker, doctor or nurse etc. to support your application
- ➤ Make sure to include the required documentary evidence to support your application. If you don't, the processing of your application will more than likely be delayed
- ➤ Make a photocopy of the application form and of any additional documentation or correspondence
- ➤ Make sure the address to which you are sending the form is correct
- ➤ If you send the application by post, register the letter. If delivering by hand, get a receipt
- ➤ Follow up your application by phoning the relevant department within a week to check that it has arrived. When calling, always have your reference number, PPS number, date of birth, address etc. to hand
- ➤ Ask for an approximate date as to when a decision is likely to be made on your application
- ➤ When in contact by phone always get the name of the person with whom you spoke. Write this down and also make a note of the date of your conversation and what was said. If a friend or

relative is assisting you with phone calls, make sure they have your documentation, reference number, PPS number, date of birth and address etc. before they make the call

➤ If phoning the Department of Social Protection or Medical Card Section, give yourself plenty of time as it can frequently take a long time for calls to be dealt with

Financial hardship

If you do not have private health insurance or a medical card, you will be liable for up to €750 per calendar year for combined inpatient and outpatient charges. However, you can apply for a waiver of these charges under Health (Amendment) Act 2005 4(b)(4) on the grounds that to pay the charges would cause undue financial hardship. Where the financial hardship is directly as a result of having cancer, you may be able to get some assistance from a variety of charitable organisations. You should discuss this with your social worker or your specialist nurse. The Money Advice and Budgeting Service (MABS) can also offer advice and assistance with budgeting. They are contactable at lo-call 1890 283438 (9.00 a.m. to 8.00 p.m. Monday to Friday) or by e-mail at helpline@mabs.ie

———◆———

PART TWO

PERSONAL ACCOUNTS

This section contains personal information about treatment for and recovery from mouth, head and neck cancers written by people who have been through treatment. The information is not intended to be prescriptive, and should not be treated as such. What works for one person does not necessarily work for everyone. Always consult your medical team before changing your treatment in any way.

———•———

CANCER OF THE PAROTID GLAND

Adrian Kennedy

I WAS A FIT 53 YEAR old in 2006. I had always looked after my health, although I wasn't fanatical about it. I cycled at least 20 kilometres most days and hiked in the mountains almost every weekend. I never smoked or drank alcohol and I grew up on a vegetarian diet. I had a general medical check-up every year and was advised that I was very healthy for my age and size.

I noticed a small lump appear just under my ear in early 2006. It was located between the end of my jawbone and the point where the lower part of the ear joins the head. At first I thought it was a large hive. The lump increased in size as the weeks passed and it became somewhat painful. By the end of February it had grown to the size of a pea and I decided it was time to see a doctor. At first my GP thought it was a cyst and he decided that we should keep an eye on it. However, by late March the lump had become more painful and I returned to my GP. He referred me to a specialist.

The specialist took two biopsies, the results of which showed the growth to be benign. I was surprised to learn that the reason for the biopsies was to determine if any cancer was present. But as the biopsies didn't show any cancer cells, I put the notion to the back of my mind. Nevertheless my specialist recommended surgery as cysts in this area can develop cancerous cells. The operation was planned for October 2006.

The pain increased gradually over the summer months. My wife and I decided to take a holiday in September, just weeks before the operation. By the time we arrived in Grenoble, France, the pain had reached a most uncomfortable level. However, when we drove up to higher ground in the Alps, the pain vanished completely and I felt better than I had in months. We spent two weeks climbing and walking in the Alps and it was wonderful to be without pain.

October arrived and I had the operation. Within hours my specialist came to my bedside to tell me how things had gone. He was clearly distressed. He said he was not happy with what he had found and that he had taken samples and would have more detailed tests carried out. On my follow-up appointment, he informed me that a cyst in my parotid gland had been cancerous. Until that moment I had never heard of the parotid gland or of cancer in that area of the head. The parotid is a salivary gland that works to release saliva into the mouth. Saliva contains enzymes that help digest food. It also contains antibodies that help protect against infections of the mouth and throat. The parotid glands are the largest of the salivary glands and most major salivary-gland tumours begin here. My surgeon said that although the operation was quite tricky, he felt he had cut out all the cancerous cells. I was later told that my surgeon was one of the most experienced in the country and that I was fortunate he had carried out the work.

First Visit to St Luke's Hospital

Within days I was assessed by a wonderful oncologist at St Luke's Hospital in Rathgar, Dublin. He had studied the report that my surgeon had provided. He explained fully and clearly to me what was wrong with me, what needed to be done to prevent further development of the cancer, what his team would do for me, how long treatments would take, how I would feel during the treatments and what the possible side effects were.

First visit to Dublin Dental Hospital

As the cancer was in the parotid gland area, my first port of call was the Dublin Dental Hospital in November 2006. I immediately knew I was in safe hands. The consultant treated me with compassion, kindness and care and also as though we had always known each other. This level of concern and care helped me to relax, knowing I was receiving expert care. I had a visual and X-ray inspection of my teeth, gums, and my mouth and jaw structure. The consultant explained clearly to me what the parotid gland is and its function. The surgery had effectively killed the gland on the affected side of my face, leaving only the remaining healthy glands to produce the necessary saliva. She mentioned that if radiotherapy was employed to 'kill off' the cancerous cells, it was most likely that I would develop a dry mouth unless the remaining salivary glands over-produced to compensate.

The dental team was wonderful. They explained that before any radiotherapy could take place, my teeth and gums had to be in good order, even if this meant removing any weak or decayed teeth. Unfortunately I had to have one molar removed, one that was quite stubborn. As I was leaving the hospital that day, the consultant mentioned to me that as time passes it is very likely that I would forget the year in which all this happened. Looking back after six years, I agree fully with this, because as I write this I have to dig deeply into my memory.

Second visit to St Luke's Hospital

Everything seemed to be moving very quickly and a couple of days after my visit to the Dental Hospital I was back in St Luke's. My oncologist explained that the most effective course of treatment would be radiotherapy. Radiotherapy is a treatment for cancer that uses penetrating beams of high-energy X-rays on the affected area of the body. He explained quite clearly to me the treatment process and gave me an estimate of the number of treatments I would need. He explained that my head would be digitally mapped so that the radiographer would be able to distinguish the healthy cells in my head and avoid them during treatment, directing the beams of radiation directly at the cancer cells. I was fascinated to hear that this level of accuracy could be achieved. It is wonderful that technology has advanced to allow this.

Third visit to St Luke's Hospital

Within days I was introduced to the team that would assist me with my recovery. An evening was arranged with the radiographers and nursing staff, so I could ask questions about my cancer treatment. I was brought into the radiotherapy room where the treatment process was clearly explained.

A mask to cover my face had to be made.[1] The purpose of the mask is to fix the patient's head to the treatment table. Before they begin the process of making the mask, a release agent is applied to the face. A release agent is similar to petroleum jelly. I recommend bringing a spare top and wearing old clothes because, although the radiographers are careful and use covers to protect your clothes, the process can be a bit messy because dental plaster and water are used to make the mould for the mask. The wet dental plaster is applied to the face in layers and is reinforced with bandaging. The plaster will get quite warm on the face but this is normal. Although quite warm, it is not enough to cause burns. In fact it is quite a pleasant experience and one should relax and enjoy the warming sensation.

When the mould is taken from one's face, a positive image of the face is

---

1. This type of mask, which entailed two hospital visits, is no longer used.

then cast from the mould and from this positive another mould is taken. Using this second mould, the technicians then cast a synthetic perspex mask to which immobilisation clamps are fitted. These clamps will then be used to attach the mask firmly to the treatment table during the patient's radiotherapy treatments. Each mask is unique and conforms exactly to a specific patient's face.

Before my treatments commenced, a series of computerised tomography (CT) scans were taken of my head. These use special X-rays designed to pinpoint the area that needs treatment. The procedure took only ten minutes to complete. The results of the scans were then used to place reference marks on my mask so that the radiographers could plot the treatment beams.

Fourth visit to St Luke's Hospital

Four weeks after my mask was completed and the CT scans were done, I was X-rayed with my mask in place in order to verify the markings and to place additional marks on the mask. These additional marks on the mask would later be used to correctly position my head for the treatment.

Fifth visit to St Luke's Hospital

I was called for my radiotherapy treatment a week later. It was wonderful to know that my treatment was now getting underway, and so quickly too, considering I had received my diagnosis just weeks previously. It was fortunate that I had visited the treatment room on my previous visit to the hospital; otherwise I would have been surprised at how dark the room is and how large the radiography projection unit is. I was warmly welcomed by two radiographers. They briefly reminded me of the procedure and handed me my treatment schedule card. The card indicated the number of treatments I was to have and the dates on which I would receive them.

I was given a radiation stent so that my healthy teeth and gums were protected from stray radiation. This stent was to be inserted in my mouth every time I underwent radiation to protect the healthy parts of my mouth and the enamel on my teeth from radiation. I was then introduced to my new mask and they confirmed that the reference on it was mine. A radiographer carefully fitted my mask to my face, making sure I felt comfortable in it. A gum and tooth stent was specially made by the Dental Hospital on my previous visit to match the structure of my mouth. I inserted my mouth stent while I was assisted onto the treatment table. I lay down facing the projector and infrared beams were used to position my head correctly for the projected beam. When correctly lined up, my mask was clamped to the table, securing my head so that no beams of radiation would stray into healthy parts of my body. Infra-red beams were once again checked and when everyone was satisfied and I was comfortably secure, the radiographers left the treatment room and went into the control room to carry out my treatment.

Lying there on my own, staring up at the projection beam, I never once felt alone because I knew the team were watching me through a closed-circuit television camera fitted to the projection beam unit. In addition there was a kind of intercom that allowed two-way communication. I was also given a trigger to hold during my treatment. I could use the trigger if I felt panicked or unwell, or if I felt I might sneeze.

It was interesting to listen to the movements of the projector above my head and to see the movement of the various lenses. Like most things in life, I soon got used to the routine and would almost nod off to sleep during my treatments. Because of this, I had to be careful after a session in case I might fall, as I sometimes had slight dizziness when I got up from the treatment table.

I had treatment daily for 35 days and as the weeks of treatment progressed, my ear and the side of my face got quite burnt, akin to sunburn. Blistering occurred and I gradually lost my beard (which, incidentally, never grew back). My wife was a huge support to me and dressed my very sensitive burns and blisters. I followed strictly the instructions given by the nursing staff and applied a special skin cream called Flamazine 1% and used Neugel for my mouth on a regular basis after treatment had finished. Without this support and treatment, I am sure the healing of my skin would not have been as successful.

As my cancer caused the loss of a parotid gland, my saliva count decreased quite a lot during the treatment period. Again, the nursing staff at St Luke's helped me by giving me a spray bottle containing a fluid that works as a saliva substitute. I was advised by them to rinse my mouth on a regular basis (a minimum of four times daily and particularly after every meal and snack) using a weak solution of bicarbonate of soda (bread soda) in tepid water. I was also advised to eat natural yoghurt to help prevent oral thrush (see Medical Terms).

Following my radiotherapy treatment, I underwent a number of magnetic resonance (MRI), CT and positron emission tomography (PET) scans. I continue to have an MRI scan annually.

Second visit to Dublin Dental Hospital

Quite soon after my radiotherapy commenced I was back at the Dublin Dental Hospital for monitoring. The consultant advised an oral-hygiene routine. I was told to use a special high-fluoride toothpaste daily to strengthen my teeth and prevent decay. I was shown how to apply this gel/paste using plastic dental trays. This routine also involved lining the inside of my fluoride tray/gum shield with a gel called Corsodyl. This gel is a chlorhexidine digluconate, which is an antiseptic. The gum shield was pushed over my teeth and allowed to stay in place for a matter of minutes, to allow the chemicals in the gel to react with my teeth. It was important not to rinse my mouth when the shield was removed.

I found this exercise to be the worst part of my treatments, and that includes the dressing of my burnt wounds, because the taste and texture of the gel made me want to vomit. In addition to the gel treatment, the consultant advised that I use only soft-grade toothbrushes in future. Flossing and the daily use of interdental brushes were strongly encouraged and soon became part of my normal routine.

For the first couple of years I underwent six-monthly check-ups at the Dublin Dental Hospital. I was advised on oral cleaning techniques and a special gum shield was made so that I could cover my teeth while sleeping, because I had developed pain in my gums due to grinding my teeth while asleep. However, I soon overcame that problem and was able to sleep again without the shield after a few weeks.

A disaster happens

A disaster happened soon after the completion of my radiotherapy. My family took me to lunch to celebrate the completion of my treatment. A strange sensation came across the side of my face during the meal. I knew by the looks on the faces of my family that something strange had occured. Looking in the mirror in the washroom, I was shocked to see that one side of my face had collapsed. My eye drooped badly and there were tears running down that side of my face. The side of my mouth also drooped quite badly, leaving me with slurred speech. I called my oncologist and he saw me immediately.

The oncologist explained that I had developed a condition like Bell's palsy and that this sometimes happens after major surgery to the part of my face from where the tumour was removed. I was referred to an eye specialist but he couldn't offer me much hope. He explained the reason for the constant tears was that the tear-duct, which functions as a drainage system for the eye, was now paralysed. He checked my eyesight and fortunately my vision was okay. As the slightest breeze in my eye would cause a flood of salty tears, I was forced to always wear spectacles outdoors. In addition I had to carry a wad of soft tissues with which to dry my face every few minutes. I looked quite dreadful and avoided looking at myself in mirrors. I felt so sorry for my family and friends who had to look at me. However, after a few months, my face miraculously readjusted and the tear duct also returned to normal.

Support

You may ask how I got through all this mess. The simple answer is family, medical experts and friends. My wife and children were simply marvelous. They were pillars of strength. I know they worried about me quite a lot but not once did they show this to me. My wife in particular walked each step of the way with me. She attended every hospital and clinic visit with me. She discussed my medical problems and treatments with the medical staff. She dressed my ugly burns and wounds, but most importantly she gave me the encouragement and strength to overcome my illness. She is still travelling with me on my cancer journey and will arrive with me at the destination, whenever that happens. The medical teams were and still are wonderful. Support was offered to me from every quarter but luckily I was able to cope and I accepted my medical condition as soon as I knew the facts.

Changes

I found my saliva level could dry up at any time and I carried sugar-free chewing gum with me to help. Parts of my face were left paralysed but this I assume is due to the surgery and not the radiotherapy treatments. I have tinnitus in the affected ear but I have learned to accept it, so I don't notice it unless I listen for it. The physical structure of my inner ear is slowly changing in shape. This causes a regular build-up of earwax. Weekly application of oil helps.

Food and diet

Soon after radiotherapy commenced, my sense of taste changed drastically for a broad range of foods. Foods I never liked became interesting, while some foods I had previously enjoyed became unpleasant to eat. I noticed the flavour of salt in nearly all processed foods and sweets. Even now, more than six years later, my experience of certain flavours has remained different from what it was before the cancer.

I was a vegetarian prior to treatment, but my diet was well balanced, so no changes were required. I never drank alcohol either and this helped.

Life today

Today I feel great. Apart from the inability to grow a beard on one side of my face and a very slight scar on my neck, I feel the same, health-wise, as before 2006.

———•———

Hannah O'Driscoll

IN SEPTEMBER 1999 I WAS diagnosed with breast cancer, had a lumpectomy, followed by radiotherapy, and made an excellent recovery.

Early in 2008, I noticed a small lump behind my left earlobe. There was no pain or discomfort. In June 2008 I sought medical advice.

In January 2009, an ear, nose and throat (ENT) consultant diagnosed parotid swelling/lump.

That March, following fine needle aspiration and an MRI scan, the lump was removed and examined. The pathology report stated that the lump was a mucoepidermoid carcinoma – a small, malignant, localised, high-grade tumour. I had not considered that a lump that seemed so insignificant could have so many consequences.

The treatment

Thirty-nine sessions (ten minutes each day over seven weeks) of intensity modulated radiotherapy (IMRT).

Prepration for treatment

The surgeon was very informative about my diagnosis and the proposed treatment. When an oncologist took over my care, he confirmed everything the surgeon had told me. I found this very reassuring. The preparation for the IMRT was as follows:

➤ Attend the Dental Hospital and follow the doctor's instructions. I had two extractions, impressions for trays were taken and I received a copy of the very informative booklet *Therapeutic Radiation and Oral Health,* which proved invaluable

➤ Visit my regular dentist

➤ Have another MRI scan and a CT scan

➤ Attend at the radiotherapy clinic of the hospital where the IMRT was to be administered. A mask was to be prepared specially for me (each mask is individual). Calculations were carried out and simulations were made and sent to the US for planning. Then the mask was made in Dublin

When all the preparations were completed, I was called by the radiotherapy clinic for a 'dummy session' of IMRT. It was like a rehearsal for 'the big day' when the IMRT would start. I was taken through everything that was going to happen with the IMRT.

I was taken to the changing room. I undressed to the waist and put on a special gown. I was shown around one of the radiotherapy rooms and shown the machines. I lay on the table and the mask was fitted and fixed. The fit of the mask was relevant as moving my head during the treatment would mean that the rays would not be directed at the appropriate target (the parotid gland, in my case). I was told I could choose to have music or not and could bring my own CD if I wished. The treatment began a few days later. That's when the daily routine started.

Challenges

The diagnosis was a bolt out of the blue. I did not even remotely suspect that the lump behind my earlobe was anything other than a simple swelling that would disappear in its own time. My GP's assessment had reassured me further. But having already survived breast cancer helped me to be positive. The breast and parotid cancers were not related and this was a great source of comfort to me.

Getting to and from therapy

My husband drove me to and collected me from my therapy sessions most days. This was my preferred way of travel, but of course it wasn't always possible. On occasion my daughter collected me or I took a taxi one way. Unusually for me, I needed the routine, the same thing every day: same mode of transport, dropped at the same spot and collected there again. It was a short journey (about 15 minutes). Gradually I settled in to the routine.

During my treatment, I didn't want to meet anyone or socialise outside my immediate family. Also, I avoided the telephone as much as was possible. I felt out of my depth and that my life revolved around the treatment. My focus was to sustain myself and to complete the course of IMRT. It was very unusual for me to be so self-centred.

Fatigue

This was not a big problem as I took bed rest every day after the treatment.

Pain and pain management

I was able to cope with the discomforts. I followed all the suggestions and advice given by my health specialist as much as I could, and they let me know that there was help if and when I needed it. I felt that they were listening, even when, with hindsight, my questions must have seemed unreasonable.

Yoga

Yoga is a big part of my life and I found it to be a great 'friend' to me after the diagnosis, during the preparations (MRI scans etc.) and during my treatment. Prayer and trust also helped tremendously. I availed of the cancer support services in the hospital during and after my treatment. I believe in a holistic approach to healing.

Food and diet

Some foods tasted different. For example I stopped eating chocolate and lost my desire for sweet food in general. This was very convenient as it helped my teeth.

I saw a dietitian at the hospital. This was part of my routine care as it was important that I should not lose weight (otherwise the mask would not fit well). The dietitian encouraged me to eat all manner of food to maintain my weight!

Dry mouth

I experienced dry mouth. At first I didn't know what it was, even though I had been warned that it would happen. The usual advice worked for me: bring a small bottle of water everywhere, keep a glass of water on my bedside locker and another glass to hold the rinsing of my mouth before I sipped fresh water. Having the water and rinsing glass beside my bed helped to keep me in sleep mode.

Anxiety

Yes, there was a lot of it. It took a lot of mindfulness to keep that in check. Again my health professionals were very helpful. They always listened and reassured me where possible. I gradually learned to live one day at a time and even moment to moment.

Books and CDs I found helpful

- ➤ *The Power of Now* by Eckhart Tolle.
- ➤ *A New Earth: Awakening to Your Life's Purpose* by Eckhart Tolle
- ➤ Seamus Heaney's poetry
- ➤ *Moments of Stillness* by Sister Stan. Open a page at random and get inspiration!

When holding a book is tiring, listening to a CD is great. *A New Earth – Awakening to Your Life's Purpose* by Eckhart Tolle is available as an audiobook or you could listen to your favourite music.

Private outcomes

- ➤ I am better able to appreciate each new day and each part of my day
- ➤ I am more determined to *do* something about fulfilling my dreams
- ➤ I 'don't sweat the small stuff' so much
- ➤ I walk every day, if possible
- ➤ I'm more willing to try new things with a nothing-to-lose attitude
- ➤ I look for the positive in situations

———•———

Ian Quigley

I WAS ORIGINALLY DIAGNOSED WITH non-Hodgkin's lymphoma in 2006. At the time I was confused as the doctors were unsure about the diagnosis, mainly because it was purely cutaneous in four localised areas on my left shoulder. So the first time I appreciated that I had cancer was at my six-month check-up, after having chemotherapy and radiotherapy. I mistakenly thought that a cancer could be benign. I think not worrying about having cancer was a great help.

In 2010 I found a lump in my neck. It didn't go away, so after a few months of 'It's probably harmless' from one doctor, the second one sent me for tests. The syringed fluid 'looked okay' and the lump, removed surgically, also 'looked okay'. Again, it wasn't until after the main treatment was carried out and the cancer had been removed that I was diagnosed. I went on to have radiotherapy, which I'd had before, in 2006, so it really didn't concern me.

What surprises me? Sometimes, actually, nearly all the time, I forget that I ever had cancer. I tell my friends and co-workers and they say, 'Oh, that's why you have a scar on your neck.' You'd never guess.

I never really had too many problems with the treatments. I had to keep myself out of the sun while I had radiotherapy burns. I was back in work just over a week after having my parotid gland removed. The surgery did hurt like heck for a few weeks and I couldn't look over my shoulder when reversing the car for about two months.

I don't see much point in worrying about cancer. The media probably over-hypes it. That's not to say it's not serious; it is. I don't know why I got cancer twice and, to be honest, I don't very much care why. I don't wonder why I have good or bad luck or why it's raining today. It's just life, and there's not much you can do about it. Choosing to be happy, or at least to see the bright side, is something I can do.

Suggestions

I think it's a good idea to focus on more personal or specific cases rather than on statistics and numbers. To me '95 per cent of patients survive cancer X' is pretty meaningless because I'd focus on the 5 per cent who don't make it. I think my 'I had cancer, I got over it and I'm totally healthy(ish)' story is more meaningful to people in a similar position. They can probably relate to it.

Food and diet

I eat and drink pretty much normal stuff. If anything, I probably had too many 'sympathy' take-away curries and Chinese meals.

————•————

Ann Allen

LOOKING BACK I THINK I was in shock. The lump in my neck that was 85 per cent likely to be nothing, turned out to be a squamous-cell carcinoma of the salivary gland – i.e. cancer – with neck lymph-node involvement, and it was already spreading. I told family and friends with a real sense of detachment. The ENT consultant was already making plans for neck surgery to remove lymph nodes. Radiotherapy afterwards was a given, and maybe chemotherapy. A few weeks previously I had been skiing, and had no sense of what was coming. What else could I do? I just went with it. Everyone rallied round, trying to be supportive. 'You are strong, but don't be afraid to be angry, or worried, or to cry,' they all said. The truth is that I felt nothing!

Over the next six months, I went from being a fit, healthy, lively individual to being scrawny, scarred, exhausted, nauseous, in pain, anxious and half bald. Food became a dirty word. Nearly eight weeks of radiotherapy, with chemotherapy once a week for six of those weeks, will do that to you. Each day I woke up and my first thought was, *Here we go again*. I was given a target intake of 2,000 calories a day. I struggled to hit 1,500. The threat of tube feeding hung over me. My dietitian, who had boundless enthusiasm, kept me going.

It didn't stop once the treatment was over and it wasn't until nearly three weeks after treatment finished that I first attempted solid food, having resorted to an exclusively liquid diet for the five previous weeks. I never thought I would be so nervous about eating a sausage!

It's just coming up to 18 months since I finished treatment. I can't believe that I have come so far. My positives are still sometimes tempered with negatives. I've made it through but I miss my scar-free neck. I can take pleasure in food again, except bread, pastries, red meat, chunky food, chocolate, sweet drinks, cakes, fruit without yoghurt and anything not smothered in sauce! I drink lots of water, but I wake up with my mouth dry as a board during the night. My teeth get much better care than before, but I have to do this drag of a routine every night to protect them.

I feel lucky to be here and healthy but the worry still lingers there in the back of my mind. I have been shown amazing support, kindness and patience on my cancer journey. I have been blessed with a partner who has been my rock through it all. He even made the supreme sacrifice of eating all that delicious high-calorie food when I couldn't manage it! I hope I never have to go through this again. But for now, I'm alive and I can't ask for more than that.

Food and diet

We are no chefs in my house, so no Cordon Bleu suggestions!

- ➤ Getting back onto solid foods, I found sausages were great, a bit spicy, cut into small pieces, with lots of beans for moisture

- ➤ Omelette was another easy food to make and eat. Initially, I couldn't have much in it, but I added things like onion and ham over time

Suggestions

- ➤ Have a ball before you start treatment. You will lose serious weight, so why not live a little before it gets crappy. I ate and drank without guilt and piled on the pounds. It probably saved me from having to be tube fed towards the end of my treatment[2]

- ➤ If you can afford it, stay off work as long as you can (at least three months after treatment finishes)

- ➤ I did a mindfulness course at St Luke's Hospital which I found very helpful

- ➤ Accept that recovery takes time and is different for everyone

---

2. Check with your dietitian before making changes to your diet.

> ➤ The ARC Centre on South Circular Road in Dublin offers amazing support. The classes on relaxation are great.

———◆———

Edward Naessens

The last thing I expected

IT STARTED WITH A TINY bump and a strange zing in my cheek. I was 24 and I didn't want to make a fuss. Who wants to be called a hypochondriac? There was a tiny lump tucked under my earlobe, and the zingy shock happened whenever I ate things like citrus or chewing gum. I was more curious than concerned about my symptoms. They seemed odd but not threatening and they were so subtle that I thought they were barely worth mentioning.

It got a bit annoying so I mentioned it to the GP I had at that time. She wasn't alarmed and suggested it would clear up. I was otherwise healthy and I looked after myself reasonably well. The worst medical problem I'd had up to that was nosebleeds, which were simple to sort out. I thought this blockage would be the same. Months later it was still there, so I mentioned it to the GP again and suggested that it could be a problem with my salivary gland. She dismissed this suggestion and said the bump under my earlobe was too far back to have anything to do with the salivary glands.

She arranged for me to see a consultant and this got investigations going. A few months later a post-op biopsy detected cancer … in my salivary gland. I have a nasty habit of being right about things I wish I was wrong about.

After surgery I was told things were fine, that it was sorted and I had nothing to worry about.

Years later a recurrence was discovered. I was even more shocked. It was a rare head and neck cancer. My point is that being stunned, shocked, terrified and bewildered is all par for the course. The second time round it was far more serious and complicated. I got second opinions in New York and London, and eventually I switched to another hospital.

Finally, after a long course of treatment and recovery, I pulled through. The approach I took, and still take, is simple: focus on what works, avoid what doesn't. Flapping, panicking, worrying, feeling helpless and morose are all very understandable reactions. They're also quite useless.

A better approach is to reach out and get advice and support. Stick to what will increase your chances of survival and recovery. Focus on what is going to get you the best result possible in the situation. Going into treatment you may hear that you will be incapacitated in one way or another. In my case I was facing facial paralysis, deafness, and loss of balance. It is never easy to accept these things. Yet if you think about it, ordinary people do extraordinary things after huge setbacks. There is always somebody worse off than you, somebody who has been through or is going through worse. There are always worse things that could have happened. I really found that looking to tougher circumstances faced by others gave me perspective. I remember reading Anthony Beevor's excellent book *Stalingrad*, an account of the appalling conditions endured by both Russian and German troops during WWII. Counting your blessings can sometimes be hard, but it really works.

'There is nothing either good or bad, but thinking makes it so.'

(Hamlet)

Having come through treatment I faced a new problem, namely the fear of a recurrence. It was tough trying to rebuild knowing I may well be faced with more destruction. If I wake up in the morning with a pain in my jaw, I immediately think the worst. This is where psychology comes into play. You have to take your self-talk in hand. Your mind can terrify you into depression and inertia. I strongly recommend some form of cognitive behavioural therapy (CBT), which will give you a script to have ready for those horrible anxiety attacks.

Rest is important. Self-talk tends to be negative when you're tired or a bit under the weather. Often a good night's sleep or a slow walk in nature can make a big difference to mood.

The support I got from people was great. Some don't know what to do or what way to approach you, but that's fine. I was positively surprised by how people simply wanted to help.

I'm trying to find the balance between telling you that not alone can you survive cancer but you can thrive, and, on the other hand, letting you know that it will be tough. In fact several psychological research studies point to the effective twin-track approach of *a.* knowing you can do X (where X is a big challenge) and *b.* understanding that achieving your X will be difficult.

There are big challenges to overcome, problems to be solved and mental games to be played. As I see it, one of the big problems is separating what you can control and what you can't control. No two cancers are the same and no two people are the same. Therefore there is the distinct possibility that taking control of the things you *can* control could make a difference in terms of outcome. The more steps you can take to benefit your physical and mental health, the more you can improve your outcomes.

To google or not to google

There are two schools of thought on this. I don't think there's any harm looking at information as long as your focus is to improve your chances of a better outcome. Though my cancer was rare, I found a webpage for it, run by people with the condition. It made for difficult reading because it was maudlin. Feeling sad is all fine and well but in terms of empowering you to swing the odds in your favour, I don't think it works. The only reason to spend time reading up on any condition is to find something that does something positive for you. People 'catastrophising' or sharing how sad they are about their condition is, of itself, pointless. Sharing solutions and ideas, however, is really worthwhile for both the reader and the writer.

Take ownership of your treatment. I was given an over-the-counter medication for nausea. It wasn't working so I asked my GP for a prescription for a drug that had worked for me before. One member of the oncology team felt it wasn't necessary, but I was the one with the nausea and his solution wasn't working. You don't have to agree on everything with your oncology team. Obviously the big stuff like the surgery, radiotherapy (RT), computerised tomography (CT) are things you probably want to leave to the highly trained. I don't believe in DIY oncology – the electricity bill for doing an MRI scan at home is ridiculous! But things like what foods you like, or what pain relief works better for you, are areas where you should feel free to express a preference.

I have to be careful about what I am about to say. But I feel I have more than earned the right to say it given the mixed bag of experiences I have had with medical staff and institutions. A white coat or a uniform do not an expert make. Not all specialists are that special. Not all nurses are Florence Nightingale. The standard of care I experienced was for the most part world-class, but some was appalling. Don't be afraid to report or stand up to substandard or rude treatment. Your loyalty should be to no one but yourself and those who care for your best interests. You may be frail, sick, low on patience, but you always deserve professional care. If any abuse is going to happen it's most likely to happen when you are vulnerable. Make sure your support network is aware of this. For the most part you will meet professional and friendly staff but do not rule out meeting the negligent, the careless, the burnt-out, and the Nurse Ratcheds. Notify your support network, make a fuss, and take no prisoners if needs be.

Dental health

Good dental habits are essential. Head and neck cancer treatment generally has an impact on teeth. I quickly decided that the days of lax dental routines were over. Radiation, for example, lowers bone density. Dry mouth and/or reduced saliva mean less protection for your teeth. And your teeth will need all the help they can get. Habits take a week of effort to form, and after that they make life a lot easier. So go for it – awaken the obsessive compulsive within; it will make life easier.

What seem like healthy drinks are not always so good for your dental health. If you drink fruit juice or eat acidic fruit, make a point of rinsing and washing it down with a glass of water. Do not brush your teeth until half an hour has passed because acidic fruit juices can temporarily soften the surface of the tooth. The same goes for red wine. I like a glass of red wine or two (strictly measured at 125 mls) but again it is hard on the teeth. Do get an electric tooth brush and use interdental brushes; they both do a good job. See your dental hygienist and learn not to be too terrified of their criticism –they really are trying to help (I think!).

Food and diet (or: get a big dinner plate)

If appetite becomes a problem there are a few ways to improve things. Here are just a couple for starters. When your appetite is low one of the ways to play a little trick on your mind is to put a regular portion on a bigger plate. It's an effective illusion. Also, look through appetising cookbooks. This works to stimulate your mind positively when your appetite is low.

Don't be fooled by thoughts of finality

If you're feeling isolated and that all those well-meaning people around you don't understand what you're going through, then you are generally right. The experience of having a life-threatening condition is literally unimaginable. The fear of death and what might happen before you shuffle off your clogs is terrifying. Don't avoid those thoughts – you can't. However, when you indulge them, and I mean really go for it, you'll discover that they are quite literally a dead end, a cul-de-sac. There is nothing more you can do with them. They go nowhere. Just realising their pointlessness is a good enough reason to indulge them. When you get to that point you can focus on adapting to your new situation and finding ways to meet the challenges that come with a cancer diagnosis.

The truth is that with time, after a setback, your mood and happiness improve. Researchers refer to this as 'mean reversion'. University of Massachusetts researchers suggest that within a year after a lottery win or becoming paraplegic, people who experience these major events return to the same level of happiness they enjoyed prior to the events. It is possible to be happy and live a good life even with the concerns that come with a diagnosis. I like to think of it this way: even without cancer I would have had other things to worry about. I like to think that at the very least the quality of my worries has improved.

Books, websites and CDs I found helpful

➤ *50 Essential Things to Do When the Doctor Says It's Cancer* by Greg Anderson. Lots of useful advice and tips from a man who went through cancer

➤ *Succeed* by Heidi Grant Halvorson. This is a good read on the science of motivation. What actually works and what our common sense tells us will work are often at odds. Prepare for some surprising information

➤ I like the work of Martin Seligman but in particular his CD training course *Learned Optimism*. It is the type of exercise that is worth returning to a few times. Again, it will surprise you with how the scientific studies of happiness contradict our common sense view of how the mind works and what makes us tick.

➤ Mood Gym (www.moodgym.anu.edu.au). My current GP recommended this to me. It is a good introduction to CBT. Be patient with it, as it is designed for teens and college students but the underlying content is useful for all.

Conclusion

Cancer is a horrible thing to happen. Head and Neck cancers come with more complexity as treatment can affect speech, hearing, eating, and facial expression. But the options and treatment methods have improved and for every problem there is usually more than one solution. It will often be tough but you can do it. Your job is to figure out the best way for you.

———•———

CANCER OF THE EAR

Charles Dobbyn

2011 IS THE YEAR I will never forget. A water blister appeared on my ear, which was very sore. My GP sent me to hospital, where they cut part of my ear off. When they took the stitches out they said everything was okay.

Four months later a lump appeared between my ear and my eye. This caused pain and as time went by I became dependent on painkillers. I went back to my GP and he sent me back to hospital. They did a biopsy, which proved positive, so they decided to send me to St James's Hospital. When the ENT consultant saw the X-rays I was admitted straight away. My wife asked him what were my chances and he said 50/50 if I had the operation, none if I didn't. This was a shock I didn't expect. He said they didn't know how far the cancer had gone in.

I had to wait two weeks for the operation, which was a nightmare. Depression set in, lying there day after day. I kept thinking of my loved ones who I may never see again. That was hard. Finally operation day came. They took the ear and had to do a lot more work around the area. After a few weeks they sent me home for a while. I went to St Luke's for radiotherapy for six and a half weeks. During my stay I lost my appetite, and three stone in weight, due to the metallic taste in my mouth, but after a couple of months I started to eat regularly again.

The challenge
To live a long and happy life.

Pain
I have very little.

Eating
Small amount of discomfort due to stiffness of the jaw and reduced opening.

Disfigurement
Doesn't bother me. I'm the same person but I look a bit different. When you see me, you know what to expect the next time.

Family
Without my wife and family I would not be here today. They are my life and my challenge is to be there with them. I also have four very good friends and great neighbours.

Dental problems

Very few. Each dental appointment was a pleasure to attend at the Dublin Dental Hospital. They were brilliant, which I am grateful for.

Silver lining

Every story should have a silver lining. Mine is, I'm still here.

Suggestions

Don't give up.

Final thoughts

I think of the doctors and nurses who looked after me in both hospitals, especially the intensive care nurses, who encouraged me to fight on. And to all the other people who were there for me, thank you all!

CANCER OF THE MAXILLA

Ben Wu

BEFORE THE CANCER WAS DIAGNOSED, my wife and I both had good jobs. We had just bought our new house together and life was good. Every year, if we were not home visiting friends and family, we would make trips abroad. In January 2008 our first child was born. She is a miracle baby, and even now as she passes her fifth birthday, I think of her as a miracle. I should have known then there is no such thing as miracles.

In June 2009 I was diagnosed with stage 2B osteosarcoma of the jaw. It is a rare type of cancer which is most commonly found in adolescence. I was nearly 42 years old when I was diagnosed with the disease. The first symptom I had was no more than a toothache. I was seen by two dentists and one specialist, had my tooth extracted and thought the pain would go. However, three or four months later the pain was still there, so I went to a specialist who took an X–ray. He reckoned it might be a salivary gland infection and he referred me to St James's Hospital. The minute the consultant saw the limited opening of my mouth and the slight swelling of my right jaw, he knew it was something more than just a salivary gland infection. He insisted I should be admitted to the hospital and stay for a CT scan, an MRI, a PET scan and a biopsy. Finally it was confirmed to be a tumour measuring around 10 cm in diameter, growing in the cavity of my right mandible (jawbone).

Because of the rapid growth of the tumour, I was told if I didn't have the surgery to remove it, I might only live for six months. When I heard this, I just wished that it was a nightmare, that someone would wake me up. Before this point, I didn't even know that mouth, head and neck cancer existed.

All of a sudden, you feel that you have no control over your own life, your own destiny. Then, before I knew it, I was in the middle of four cycles of the most intensive and gruesome chemotherapy. I almost had every single side effect you could imagine: hair loss, nausea, tiredness, constipation, fever, low white-blood-cell count, etc. Who would have expected that after all those gruesome chemotherapy sessions the tumour would show no sign of shrinking? Immediate surgery was necessary.

I was scheduled to have the surgery in October 2009. Despite several last-minute cancellations due to lack of beds in the Intensive Care Unit, the surgery took place on 15 October 2009. It was a ten-hour surgery and I woke up the following day. When I woke up, I had drips all over my body, my head and face were swollen like a balloon and I must have had more than a hundred stitches. When you add the tracheostomy they did to aid recovery ('tracky', they call it). I was pretty much like someone from a horror movie.

When my mum and my wife came up to the High Dependency Unit (HDU) to see me like this, they both just broke down in tears. I was in tears too as I knew how difficult it must be for them to see me like this. That must have been the lowest and saddest moment of my life.

Because of the 'tracky' thing I had no speech, so I had to write things down and show the nurses. Even a journey to the loo required a nurse's assistance. The physical pain could be managed by drugs, but mentally it was too much to take in. I was warned all along that after the surgery I could be quite disfigured and I couldn't bear to look at myself in the mirror for quite some time. The thought of scaring my two-year-old daughter was unbearable but luckily I was told I was not that scary and my two year old couldn't wait for me to be strong enough to hold her again.

I still remember a nun who brought me a card that had the 'Footprints in the Sand' prayer on it. It was then I realised that all this pain and the burdens caused by the Big C, all the sorrow and sadness were things I had to go through. God had always been there with me. I broke down in tears, and it was from that moment on that I had faith.

I think after two weeks in hospital I was sent home to recover. I had a speech therapist and a dietitian. Both were a great help in getting my speech and health back. Little by little my strength and health came back and the following year, 2010, I started 22 sessions of radiotherapy treatment. The purpose was to reduce the chance of the cancer cells coming back. So, after all this treatment and surgery, I thought my life could get back to normal. Again, with the constant CT scan appointments and hospital check-ups, I thought somehow that the Big C had left for ever.

I think it was around Easter when a CT scan showed the cancer was back. There was a metastasis in my right lung. Once more I was devastated by the news. Even though I was warned that it was most likely it would spread to the lung, somehow you just want to deny that it is actually happening again. Because the tumours were small, I was advised to stay put and wait and see if they had spread to other parts of the body. Also they wanted to wait till it got bigger to operate. It was even harder to take in than the first time I was diagnosed. This horrible picture of myself in the High Dependency Unit with all those drips and tubes was unbearable. *Why, why, is it me again?*

Once again I thought I had let myself down, let my family down. And I decided to seek help, to have psychotherapy. It helps to have someone there who can listen. Before I knew it I was recovering from another surgical procedure. There were no chemotherapy or radiotherapy treatments needed this time, so once again I thought I had beat this damn disease. I was sent home to recover.

In early 2012, the disease was back. This time there was another metastasis in my left lung, and in June I had another operation. My last scan showed I was clear so far.

I don't know what the future holds for me and I don't know when the disease will be back again. It has been almost four years since I was diagnosed. I've had two relapses since. Each time was hard, each time involved doubts and uncertainties, but I found myself coping with it better each time. Well, if you can't beat it, embrace it. If it doesn't kill you, it makes you stronger.

It has been an emotional ride for me and my family. I have met some very kind, compassionate people along the way, some of whom are not here anymore. But those who are still here show me such kindness and support; it's why I'm still here today.

There is always light at the end of the tunnel. Be positive, be active, and live your life to the fullest, because as a cancer survivor you don't have the luxury of time to do things later. You don't know what the next scan will show or what the consultants will say. May as well just enjoy every minute of it.

My daughter is five years old now. I thought I would never see the day, and I have set my goal higher and higher each time: to live and see her grow up. My whole cancer journey has been a tremendous experience. If I could choose, I would have asked God to take away this awful disease but not the experience.

Suggestions

➤ Use Corsodyl dental gel for your teeth and gums, BioXtra oral gel for your dry mouth and Elizabeth Arden Eight Hour Cream for your dry lips.

➤ Take up yoga or tai chi and be active.

➤ Be kind a little, live a little, love a little, And be thankful that you are still alive.

➤ Stay strong, be positive and have faith.

Conclusion

Be kind to yourself and most importantly: we are still here. I hope that one day this disease called cancer will no longer exist, or can be cured.

Edward Anthony Morrall

TO MOST PEOPLE CANCER IS a scary word but it is not always fatal, as I found out for myself. My experience started with a routine dental check-up in 2005. The dentist found a small growth on my gum and said he thought it should be checked out. I agreed and I thanked him.

I next got an appointment to see a consultant at St James's Hospital. He arranged for me to have CT scans, various tests and finally a biopsy, which showed I had cancer in my jaw. Both my wife and I were stunned as we had hoped it was something like a cyst. The consultant explained I had a cancer called ameloblastoma. It was slow-growing but it was close to my brain. I asked him if anything could be done. He said yes, but it would have to be done soon.

We came home and had a worrying few weeks until I got a call from St James's to go in that day as they had a bed for me. Meanwhile my two sons came over from England, where we used to live, and they checked out the situation with us.

After the usual pre-op preparations I had surgery on my jaw. I woke up with my head wrapped in bandages. There were tubes coming out of my nose and a hole in my throat to breathe through called a tracheostomy. I had conversations with my visitors via a writing pad.

I was in the High Dependency Unit for about ten days and then I signed myself out into the excellent care of my wife. At home you adjust your lifestyle to suit your circumstances. There were regular visits to the hospital to have a type of denture called an obturator (see Medical Terms) made for me, and to learn how to eat and drink again. My meals at home started with rice pudding and yoghurt, that type of food – easy to swallow – but I eventually got around to a proper meal: five vegetables with meat or fish.

I found it easier to swallow my food if I mashed it up and had plenty of gravy on it. People in the hospital asked me if I got depressed, as it's a problem for some people. I said not really as I'm an optimist by nature so that helps. As I see it, I had a problem, my consultant was able to fix it and I am alive!

On the downside, before the operation I played the French horn in a symphony orchestra, which I enjoyed. Not any more, but that's life.

———◆———

CANCER ON THE BASE OF THE TONGUE

Milena Venkova

AT THE TIME OF MY diagnosis I was 36, had a four year old and a six-month-old baby, and was on maternity leave from my full-time job. A lump appeared on my neck during pregnancy and I mentioned it to my GP. He said we would have to check it out if it was still there at my next appointment, but he didn't seem worried. At my next appointment the lump was still there, so he sent me for blood tests to St Vincent's Hospital.

In the meantime my baby arrived, and life was fairly busy. I worried a bit about the lump, but a recurring tooth infection seemed a plausible explanation for it. Eventually the tooth infection had to be dealt with by a specialist, so I asked the endodontist (see Medical Terms) if it could be causing the lump on my neck. He became very serious and told me to go back to my GP and ask for further tests. So I did, and when I showed him that the lump was still there, my GP literally turned green.

He immediately sent me back to St Vincent's Hospital, where I had a needle biopsy and was diagnosed with a squamous cell carcinoma at the base of my tongue. I had never heard of it before. The doctor on duty, a girl around my age, made me promise I would not look it up on the internet, and promised in return to answer any questions I had. An important lesson if you haven't been around hospitals much: ask questions!

It took eight months from my first mention of the lump to diagnosis. Partly the reason was that I was young, female and a non-smoker, and mouth cancer would be extremely unusual in my case. Another reason was that mouth cancer doesn't show on blood tests. Bad luck, really. The cancer had spread to a lymph node in my neck, and that is how it got detected. I never noticed any pain or difficulty swallowing. Basically, I was a perfectly healthy person, apart from the cancer.

The doctors' first job was to do every known test on me: MRI, PET scan, CAT scan, a biopsy under general anaesthetic. It was determined that the cancer had spread to the lymph nodes in my neck but no further, which placed me firmly at stage three. Within two weeks I had two trips to the Dublin Dental Hospital, the first one to determine what treatments my teeth would need, and the second one to extract the teeth that had serious problems. It turned out there were four of them, and I can't say I enjoyed that.

I also had a radical neck dissection – which basically means the surgeons removed the lymph nodes on the affected side of the neck. It was major surgery, but the recovery took only a week. One side effect was that a nerve that moves a muscle on my shoulder had to be severed, and this affects my shoulder to this day. I have to do exercises on a regular basis to keep my shoulder functioning, and even so I have serious muscle loss. With hindsight, a few things that seemed insignificant at the time, since they were not life threatening, turned out to be very significant with the passage of time. One was the damage to my shoulder, another was the reduced mouth opening, but more on that later.

During a three-month wait I had to try to put on as much weight as possible (not a common concern for a young woman!). Eventually I started radiotherapy combined with chemotherapy in St Luke's Hospital. Since the carcinoma at the base of my tongue was not surgically removed, to avoid damage to my tongue, it had to be treated exclusively with radiotherapy. That meant 35 sessions and five weekly chemotherapy sessions. I refused to have a PEG tube fitted to my stomach. My decision was quite irrational – it is a minor surgery compared to the one I had been through – but I was convinced I could get through without it. For the first three to four weeks of treatment the side effects weren't noticeable. The chemotherapy meant I was bursting with energy for three days of the week and tired the rest, but nothing particularly dramatic.

My mouth and throat were getting sore, but with the help of standard painkillers I could eat soft food, yoghurt and ice cream. Eventually I was put on morphine, and I wish someone had told me about the severe constipation it causes!

By week five I was doing well, living at home and travelling on the Luas for daily radiotherapy sessions. And then on Sunday I woke up with a high temperature and I was unable to swallow even water. On Monday back at the hospital several attempts were made to pass a tube through my nose into my stomach, but my throat was so swollen that the tube couldn't get through. Eventually it was agreed that I'd be fed and watered intravenously. Blood tests eventually showed that I had picked up a throat infection, and I had to be put on an antibiotic drip. That was the beginning of my month-long stay in St Luke's.

Once the antibiotics had worked and the swelling was down, a tube was passed through my nose for feeding. At some stage I had a drip on each hand and a tube in my nose, and I wish I'd had a picture taken! In a way being fed through a tube was a relief, because my mouth and throat weren't sore when I didn't have to swallow. I did attract a few stares on the streets on my trips out, though. Two weeks after the radiotherapy was finished I could swallow liquids again, so the tube was removed and I could go home.

Mentally, I wasn't prepared for what followed. I expected my recovery to be as quick as after the surgery, but it took a lot longer and I did indeed lose almost two stone in three to four months.

A warning: If you are on morphine, the dose needs to be reduced gradually. I didn't know that, and as a result suffered the weekend from hell once my prescription ran out.

Another warning: Do some mouth-stretching exercises in those early months after treatment. By the time I discovered I needed to do them it was too late, and the permanently reduced mouth opening makes dental treatment and hamburger eating rather difficult.

Slowly but surely the pain from swallowing disappeared, and different tastes returned. If I remember correctly, I had a problem with thrush in my mouth, which was helped by rinsing with bread soda in warm water. I quite enjoyed experimenting with food and every time I could taste something new was a small victory. It was like being a baby again. Six months after the treatment I was pretty much back to my normal diet.

It is almost exactly six years since my diagnosis. My mouth is a bit dry and I have to drink when eating to help swallowing. Otherwise, the only food I can't eat is the very spicy or the very acidic. I was worried that I wouldn't be able to taste chocolate, but that taste returned eventually, although it helps to have a warm drink with it to help it melt. A good tip is to add a bit of cream to some foods like risotto, curry etc., it makes them easier to swallow and neutralises any spice that could irritate the mouth.

My speech and general well-being were not affected, although side effects like dry mouth mean my teeth continue to need a lot of work. Together with the shoulder exercises, using fluoride gel is the only ongoing reminder of my treatment. I have a big scar on my neck and for a while I was quite conscious of it, but with time that feeling faded. I have a friend I met two years ago, and she didn't notice the scar for months until I mentioned it to her.

After the initial shock of the diagnosis, the 'why me?' and 'I am dreaming this', I went through the months of surgery and therapy feeling determined that I would put up a good fight. My family and friends rallied around, and I've never felt as loved and cared for. My mum and sisters-in-law came to stay with us to help with the children, and my husband's colleagues arranged for him to work around my treatment. One silver lining was that I found out how many great people I have in my life.

About a year after my treatment I started feeling quite anxious for no particular reason. I think that after all that attention and support, being left on my own meant my fears were starting to catch up with me. I wasn't afraid of the cancer in particular, but a phone ringing or a noise in the garden would make my heart stop. Eventually, on the advice of a friend, I started going to weekly yoga classes. I found that really helped to restore my balance, and I am still practising.

Best of luck with your treatment, and don't forget, there is life after cancer!

———◆———

Barbara Bolton

My journey began at the start of 2001. I discovered a lump on the side of my neck, below my jawbone. At first my doctor thought it could be an infected gland. But after further investigation (a biopsy) at St Vincent's Hospital, I was told it was cancer.

I got a dreadful fright. I had never heard of anyone with cancer around the neck or head area before. I was told it was at the base of my tongue, and that I needed quite a lot of radiotherapy. All this was surreal to me. I felt like I was living somebody else's life, that it couldn't be happening to me.

I started treatment at St Luke's Hospital, Dublin. My throat became sore and I also felt very tired and very cold. But with the support of my husband Billy, who was with me every step of the way and still is to this day (12 years later), I got through it.

When my treatment finished I was so tired and down in myself that I was lost, because the routine of the hospital and the fantastic support I received from the staff every day was finished. I was now at home and getting more depressed by the day. My eating habits had totally changed as my swallow had become narrower. But you can adapt quite well to this with a little imagination!

I had a setback about five years after my radiotherapy. I had a bad tooth extracted by my dentist and unfortunately developed osteoradionecrosis (see Medical Terms). If you need a tooth extracted following your radiotherapy, be sure to tell your dentist that you have had radiotherapy. You will probably be referred to a dental hospital or an oral surgeon.

I heard about a place called ARC, a Cancer Support Centre on Eccles Street (see Resources). I called them and they were so understanding and invited me in for a chat. That was the start of a wonderful learning journey for me. I learned relaxation, stress management, how to be positive and so much more. All this and my illness gave me a new confidence I never had before. I am still learning. I am very happy 12 years on. I have fantastic support from my husband and son and daughter, now 19 and 26!

I have a great support system with the Dublin Dental Hospital, which I attend every four to five months for check-ups.

If I can say one thing, it's this: try not to be frightened. Easier said than done, I know, but even in the last 12 years, there have been improvements in radiotherapy and chemotherapy. It should give you great strength to know you are in very good hands.

Suggestions for food and diet

- ➤ Mashed potatoes and vegetables are easy to eat
- ➤ Lots of gravy! I couldn't live without it!
- ➤ Fish is soft and easy to eat (no bones though!)
- ➤ Stewed fruit and yoghurts are great
- ➤ Soup is always a great stand-by

All these things are very good for you and help to keep up your strength.

I hope this helps you in some way. I wish you the very best on your journey and remember, you are not alone.

———◆———

CANCER OF THE TONGUE

Rita Kierce

'I have crossed an ocean, I have lost my tongue, from the roots of the old one a new one has sprung!'

– Grace Nicholls

LIFE WAS BUSY. I HAD just competed in the World Cross Country Championships as a member of the Irish team in Auckland, New Zealand in 1988. As you can imagine, competing internationally I had to be at the peak of my physical fitness and at the age of 29 the world was my oyster. I was enjoying the rollercoaster that was marriage and being a new mother. I married Thomas in 1989, gave birth to my first child, Sharon, the following year and my second daughter, Emer, in 1991.

Three months into my second pregnancy I developed a mouth ulcer on the right-hand side of my tongue. Eating and drinking, particularly acidic foods, became a nightmare. The pain and inflammation escalated to the point that I decided to visit my GP. Having tried numerous lotions, potions and remedies, unfortunately things did not improve but became progressively worse. It was decided to refer my case to a consultant in Limerick for further investigation.

As part of the investigations I had to have a biopsy, but because I was pregnant certain precautions needed to be taken. The samples were analysed and the results generated. The day I received my results is forever ingrained in my memory. I was at home, surrounded by my family, when I saw my GP passing the kitchen window. I was not alarmed at first, as my mother-in-law was under the care of the same GP at the time and he often did house calls.

I can still picture sitting at the end of the counter on the high stool as the news was broken in the presence of my mother and my husband. When the GP told us it was cancer, truth be told it did not register as being hugely significant, as 21 years ago the word *cancer* was not a commonly used term in the Irish vocabulary. Much of what he said that evening, although very reassuring, was lost. My focus lay solely in getting treatment, caring for my new husband and daughter, and keeping my second bundle of joy nourished and growing. That evening I felt what I can only describe as a warmth on my hand which surged through my body – a surreal calmness had washed over me and I knew deep down that I would be all right. In the following weeks there were many occasions where the tears flowed, emotions ran high and I questioned many times *Why? Why me? Why now?* But my husband, my daughter and the pregnancy kept me distracted and looking forward.

After further investigations it was decided to let the pregnancy progress and keep a close and watchful eye on my progress. I was induced in August 1991, and my second daughter Emer entered the world a month premature. I had two weeks at home with her before I was admitted to hospital for surgery to remove the tumour.

When the wounds had healed sufficiently, I had six weeks of radiotherapy treatment in St Luke's Hospital in Dublin, leaving home on Sunday night/ Monday morning and returning home on Friday evening.

Speaking and eating became difficult, and tiredness was an issue. I had to learn to enjoy soft, creamy and tasteless food. The blender became my favourite kitchen appliance. Unfortunately, as you can imagine, when you liquidise food it loses its appeal. I knew I had to keep packing in the calories to keep the engines running, so I closed my eyes and tried to visualise and conjure the textures, smells and tastes of the foods I had just blended. I became partial to milkshakes, ice cream, custard, yoghurts and anything that could be swallowed without difficulty. Nutritional supplements such as Fortisip were a blessing.

After months of altered taste because of the effect of the radiotherapy on my taste buds, the day I could taste food again was ecstasy. I jumped around the kitchen as tears of joy streamed down my cheeks.

Dry mouth was my biggest problem. Everywhere I went I had a bottle of water with me and sipped from it regularly. The saliva substitutes, mouthwashes and other products that are on the market now were not available then. Night-time was particularly difficult as my mouth was especially dry as I slept. Vaseline was good to keep my lips from chapping. I didn't favour chewing gum as I found it very difficult to chew as a result of the surgery.

Life progressed and time passed by. Weak and weary at times, I had to rest a lot. The girls were cared for by their aunts. I knew they were safe and Thomas kept the home fires burning. There weren't support groups at that time, so I relied on support from my friends and family who were wonderful, although I must admit at times I found making conversation difficult and draining. It wasn't possible to be 'sunny side up' all the time.

Christmas came and it was a welcome treat to be home and have the family together again. I knew that all was not well. My tongue began to taint and smell like rotting meat. The consultant in Limerick had done his best but it hadn't worked for me. I was referred to St Luke's Hospital again in January but this time I was isolated and underwent brachytherapy. This involved putting pins through my tongue. The pins contained radiation sources to directly treat the tongue. At this stage I was becoming fearful as they were trying their best to cure me but I was beginning to think that it was not God's plan.

Hindsight is a wonderful gift and looking back now I firmly believe my fitness and the high level of sports training stood to me. I had won many races and I was determined not to lose this one. Options were becoming scarce; my health was deteriorating and my weight declining.

Then came the most amazing thirtieth birthday present I could have ever imagined. An appointment was made for me with an ENT surgeon in the Mater Hospital. What a celebration it turned out to be. The surgeon was going to perform what I can only describe as life-saving surgery.

I had two weeks at home with my family before the surgery to prepare myself mentally, physically and emotionally. I said many goodbyes in those two weeks and my optimism was slowly wavering. My weight had dramatically dropped to a mere 6.5 stone. Morphine was keeping the pain at bay. I longed for the day of the surgery to arrive, as I knew this could be the end of the line. St Martin provided deep comfort and my mother's devotion to him provided further optimism.

Two teams of surgeons and 17 hours later, the coast was clear. A graft from my right hand was inserted to fill the gap that remained after most of my tongue tissue had been removed. A small piece of my tongue was preserved to enable speech function and to ensure that I could continue to taste food. With excellent professional help, in the form of speech and language therapists, dietitians, nurses and doctors, my fight was restored and I took on a new outlook.

For six weeks the Mater Hospital became my home. The letters, cards and well-wishes flowed and kept me optimistic. I looked forward to the post each day. Music was such a healing presence for me also. The Kilfenora and Tulla Céilí Bands rang out in the room and around the corridors as slowly my energy levels rose and I began to tap my toes gently around the room.

There were setbacks, but every journey has setbacks and in hindsight I think they allowed me more time to heal. Everyone I met on my journey was incredible, encouraging and proud of the progress I was making.

Acquiring an injury, regardless of magnitude, can be very difficult to cope with and adjust to. The many scars, or 'beauty marks' as I called them, both internal and external that remained following the surgery had to be dealt with physically, mentally and emotionally. It took some time before I could build up the courage to look in the mirror. A person's appearance and manner of speaking usually create your first impressions of them. Both my appearance and speech were altered as a result of the surgery and these were huge issues I had to confront. I needed time to come to terms with the idea before I could take the plunge and see the 'new me'.

I had to learn to speak all over again. Pronunciation and articulation of certain letters and words were difficult and still are. My neck mobility was greatly reduced, the muscles were weak and I experienced restricted mouth opening. Time and extensive physiotherapy and speech and language therapy allowed me to make great progress.

Dental problems were not something I expected to experience, but the extensive radiotherapy prior to the surgery had set me on the path to decay. The surgery made it difficult to perform simple dental procedures but with specialist care from the dental surgeons in the Dublin Dental Hospital, and from my own dentist and hygienist at home, everything was kept under control.

The many visits from Thomas, our families and friends were endless sources of joy and optimism, which kept my spirits high. As my strength and independence grew I began to take short trips into the city to familiarise myself with life outside the confines of the hospital again. An enteral feeding tube (PEG tube) was inserted into my stomach to help me to gain weight before I was discharged. In conjunction with a dietitian we drew up a meal plan that would acheive maximum calorie input, flavour and nutrition.

Homecoming arrived, and I was ecstatic. It gave me huge peace of mind to know that my consultant and his team were at the end of the phone should I have any queries, but thankfully I didn't have cause to contact them. For the first year, I returned to Dublin every month, but as the years progressed my visits to Dublin grew fewer and further between, becoming three-monthly, six-monthly and yearly visits.

After so much downtime I got to know my body and really started to listen to it. I rested well, but maybe at times I didn't concentrate enough on myself. The children, a new business and a busy family life kept my mind occupied and didn't allow me a lot of time to reflect on the magnitude of what I had just been through.

Over the years, I stole a few minutes here and there to reflect on the gravity of my situation. As support groups formed over the years I encouraged myself to attend, to listen and to talk. Sharing my story with other people helped me to appreciate the journey I had undertaken; it gave hope to others and in a way it gave me time and space to slowly grieve.

It is 21 years since a new tongue has sprung from the roots of an old one. I am now in my fifties and life has continued with its ups and downs. I walk, and enjoy the fresh air and the beautiful surroundings of my home in the Burren. I even went back to competitive running and excelled. All the milestones I reached over the years, getting through the surgery, learning to speak again, running competitively, seeing the grey hairs appear as the girls grew up and went through school and college, proved that with the right attitude, specialist intervention, a strong support network and some hard slog, anything is possible when you have the ambition and drive to succeed.

'I have the strength to face all conditions by the power that Christ gives me.'
(Phillipians 4:13)

Suggestions

> ➤ If possible give yourself treats: a hairdo, a massage, flowers, any little token to reward yourself

> ➤ Don't be afraid to ask for help; there is plenty out there and the Irish Cancer Society is wonderful

> ➤ Continue with your physiotherapy after your hospital stay. I didn't as I was (I thought) fit and wanted catch up on family time that I had lost out on with the girls

> ➤ Daily positive affirmations. My sister was wonderful with these on down days, she always came back with one to put a smile back on my face

> ➤ *Dental Care* is very important. I learned the hard way but I am still surviving, and back eating a full diet. Chocolate is one thing I cannot master but that is no harm.

Recipe

Strawberry Fortisip, and if you can get a little exercise, the fresh air is a tonic.

———◆———

Marcus Quinn

I WAS A 35-YEAR-OLD married man with a two-and-a-half-year-old son. I worked for myself. I had recently given up smoking, in May 2006. Soon after quitting I developed a mouth ulcer that wasn't clearing. I had been to the GP and was given a steroid cream. I didn't heal, so I attended the Dublin Dental Hospital, where they immediately did a biopsy on 21 December 2006, which made for a rather unpleasant Christmas. I was brought back on 2 January 2007, when I was told I had cancer. I immediately thought that this was the end.

I was told to go home, get my affairs in order and return the next morning to St James's Hospital where I would probably stay for up to two months. I had surgery to remove half my tongue and 22 lymph nodes from my neck. I had 48 stitches from under my chin to my neck and behind my ear. They did not get all the cancer cells the first time, and had to operate again. They split my chin to get the remaining cancer cells.

The muscles in my neck deteriorated, leaving me unable to swallow, so I was fed through a tube in my stomach. While in hospital I was unable to talk and had to communicate using pen and paper. I had radiotherapy for six weeks. I have had a lot of speech therapy and thankfully I'm 98 per cent back to full speech now. Throughout my stay in hospital and afterwards I worked daily doing exercises the speech therapist had given me; some of these I still do every day.

I attended St Luke's Hospital daily for radiotherapy. My wife accompanied me at the beginning and thereafter I drove myself. I was extremely tired during treatment. I was given pain relief but I also went for acupuncture, which I found helped. I was told I would probably need the feeding tube during radiotherapy but I was determined not to need it and I didn't in the end. I had to learn to swallow again. My mouth still gets stiff. My initial fear was of death, but although I was very anxious while in hospital, I don't have an ongoing fear.

I still suffer from dry mouth at night and use Biotene, which I find very helpful. I am back to normal despite everything, and alive.

———— ◆ ————

Lionel McCarthy

THAT DECEMBER OF 2001 HAD been a particularly busy one on the work front. My job was taking me to London and Paris, with early morning flights from Dublin and late-night meetings in unfamiliar surroundings. A total slave to cigarette smoking, I was having a bad time of it, what with the various smoking restrictions while travelling and the endless meetings. I felt tired and worn. I used to be fit and active but now as I walked to a meeting at Canary Wharf, with fellow workers, the Pied Piper left me behind and I was holding up progress. It was an important time; why was I so tired? Never mind, I reasoned, Christmas is coming, bringing time for a well-earned rest and a battery recharge. Home with family and friends. And so it proved. Ten days of bliss!

The New Year brought with it new work challenges and new targets. The company's success would largely depend on how well my partner and I performed. But I never saw that express train coming down the tracks, never imagined the sudden diagnosis, and never anticipated the terror it would bring, the sudden realisation of my own mortality.

It was now late February and the business was growing and getting more frenetic every day. The axe fell one morning and things would never be the same again. Standing in the shower I discovered a lump at the back of my neck. I felt it and wondered who and what was this foreign invader? Why had I not noticed it before? How bad was it? Should I seek medical advice?

Well, as luck would have it, on that very Tuesday morning I had a meeting scheduled at the College of Surgeons. We were discussing a new building with the college estates staff and I hadn't attended a doctor's surgery for over ten years. So as soon as the meeting ended, I asked as casually as I could if there were any doctors around? Mercer Medical Centre turned out to be a lifeline, from that day to this.

Next was an X-ray at the Charlemont Clinic, then an appointment with a consultant at St James's Hospital. Then the biopsy a few weeks later. Then the news that surgery was required. The primary was in my mouth. I didn't have the courage to ask how serious it was, but I knew it wasn't going be a cakewalk.

Next was the surgery and the visit from the oncologist at St James's while I was an in-patient. He was very reassuring, saying, 'You're in pretty good shape, your age is on your side, but you will require radiotherapy and chemotherapy at St Luke's.' At that stage my morale had sunk. Would there be any light on the horizon?

Thank heaven, I said to myself, for those two consultants. I had head and neck cancer, I realised, but I might have a chance if I came through the treatment and followed every instruction. Just a chance!

Unbelievably, I was still smoking cigarettes up to the day of the biopsy, which proved that I had a serious problem. It hadn't struck me that there was any connection between my smoking and the dreaded lump that caused all the problems and the lesion in my mouth. Somehow, as if by osmosis, it dawned on my hollow brain that the cigs had to go! And so they did, just as soon as I arrived home from St James's. Gone and forgotten!

The radiotherapy began. A mask was made for me. Then the daily trip to St Luke's, the familiarity with fellow sufferers, and the next stage – the impact of all of this on my teeth. This of course was another big moment.

Our group of head and neck patients numbered about 40 in all and we had a very special nurse advisor, who explained it all to us. We had the good fortune to have the dentist lecture us on the critical importance of oral hygiene, and of course an appointment was arranged at the Dublin Dental University Hospital. There would be many more visits to Lincoln Place and heroic efforts by dentists and hygienists.

The direct links between a patient's lifestyle and medical and dental treatments became very apparent as the months rolled by. And so my health was turned around, from near death to happy living, thanks to the dedicated work of the combined medical and dental teams. After the biopsy, surgery, 34 radiotherapy shots, five chemotherapy sessions, 25 visits to the Dental Hospital and the lapse of five years, I had my life back, wrapped in Christmas paper, courtesy of those fabulous professionals.

One of many fond memories was that, on the work front, nobody apart from my partner, who worked with me even in St Luke's to keep the show on the road, knew that I was ill.

The dentist recommended that I use a product called Stoppers 4 Dry Mouth to help replace my lost saliva. This has worked brilliantly for me. Without it I could never do my teaching job, deliver a talk of any kind or even enjoy a conversation with friends.

So thanks a million to you all. It has been an intensive education in what it's like to be brought back from the brink.

And who says we don't have a wonderful health service?

With best wishes and grateful thanks to you all.

———•———

Suzanne O'Leary

IN 2007 AFTER HAVING MY second child, I noticed a crack or sore on my tongue. I treated it myself with a mouthwash, Bonjela etc. None of these helped. It was affecting my eating, so I went to my doctor, who said it was just an ulcer. He said it was from having the baby and being anaemic and I got a mouthwash.

I didn't do anything more about it until I went to see my dentist in 2008 and he said I would need a biopsy. At the time I was being treated in Wexford General Hospital for something else and for anaemia, and I mentioned it to them. They said they would do the biopsy. A few weeks later they told me it was fine. Later, I found out through my hospital file that it was lichen planus (see Medical Terms).

In 2010 I was still suffering. I returned to my dentist to get fillings and I also got a gumshield fitted to see if the problem was me biting my tongue at night. He also wrote a letter to Dublin Dental Hospital. (I should say that I'd seen an ad on television about mouth cancer awareness, and it ticked some boxes.)

I received a letter for an appointment in the Dental Hospital in March. By then I was nine months pregnant, so when the consultant examined me he thought it could be because of the pregnancy, or the mercury in my fillings.

So I was to come back in three months for review. I rang in September for an appointment and received one for 13 October. When the consultant looked at my tongue he immediately said, 'Biopsy, Monday.' I got a bit of a shock. I said, 'I'm back in work on Monday,' but he emphasised that I needed it done.

On the Monday I attended Dublin Dental Hospital for the biopsy. It was uncomfortable, but okay. On leaving, I was told to wait for a letter from reception about my results the following Monday. When I got this letter it had on it 'Mouth Cancer Clinic'. This was a big shock for me.

On 24 October I was brought into a room in the hospital. The first consultant came in and said he was waiting for his colleague, a maxillofacial consultant. The maxillofacial consultant arrived and examined me, then he sat beside me and held my hand and explained that I had tongue cancer. I was sitting looking at my husband holding our nearly seven-month-old baby boy. I was trying to be brave but the tears just fell. He explained it was early, which was good, and the fact that I was young was good, etc. I was petrified by the fact that it was in my mouth/face. What would this mean: speech, scarring, disfigurement, ugliness.

He explained I would need a large section of tongue removed as well as my lymph nodes. I automatically presumed everything would be done through my mouth. It wasn't till later that I realised I needed a radical neck dissection.

After talking me through everything, the consultant told me he would give me a letter explaining what would happen next. We waited in reception for this. I then went outside to ring my mam to let her know I was fine. And I was until I had to say the C word, but thank God it was raining, so you couldn't see my tears.

I can't really remember the drive back to Wexford. I think I was just in limbo, but the letter I received was good, as it explained what was happening and what the next step was.

Wednesday I was in St James's Hospital. We met a lovely head and neck support nurse and she went through everything and brought me for bloods, X-rays and medical history. Then we met the doctor and he talked with us about the procedure; he was lovely. He also let us know that we would have a clearer picture when we had the MRI/PET scan results.

We felt a little better after this visit. My mam and my husband came, which was good, because if I didn't hear something, or picked it up wrong, I asked them; and also it meant I didn't have to explain to everyone what was going on.

Friday I went to my own doctor, just to chat and get Valium and sleeping tablets. I can be very claustrophobic and the nurse recommended I get them for the MRI/PET scan. (That Friday my grandad passed away; it was a terrible time.) I then received a call for the MRI on the Tuesday, and on my way to that appointment I got a call for the PET scan for Wednesday.

The nurse had given us her mobile number, so during all of this we could call her whenever we had a question. She was great – a real rock.

We obviously had looked on Google etc. but that just gives you too much to think about and most of the stuff we read didn't apply to my situation. The following Wednesday I was brought into St James's Hospital and met the doctor to discuss my operation.

I forgot to mention, at the earlier appointment I had asked him to draw in permanent marker on my tongue what he was taking away. He had never been asked this before, but agreed. He thought it was a good thing to do, to help me to realise what would happen.

We went through everything and the consultant told me that he wouldn't need to do the neck dissection. I was delighted but felt a bit like a fraud as I had explained to everyone what I was getting done, and now they'd see nothing.

I then went to Admissions, where I had to wait to go up to the ward. At 6.00 p.m. I went up and checked in. Next a lovely nurse took all my details. She explained it was all scheduled for the morning unless an emergency came in, etc.

I asked for a sleeping tablet and tried to sleep. At 7.30 a.m. they came for me. I put on a lovely blue gown and off we went. I went to the pre-op room, met the anaesthetist and the nurse, then the consultant came in to say hi. They were all lovely.

Next thing, I woke up in recovery. A nurse beside me asked how I was. I automatically went to speak and it worked. I wasn't clear, it was very muffled and drunk-sounding but I could speak, and that's all that mattered. I'd expected nothing. Also, I had no tube in my trachea. I was there for an hour and was then transferred to the ward. Then Mam arrived and said, 'Two fingers for *yes*, one for *no*.'

I said, 'Why? I can talk!' and she filled up.

I slept most of the day, but I do remember I wanted to scrub my teeth and wasn't allowed. They did, however, give me sticks with sponges and a little water, which were heaven. I was fed through a small yellow tube connected to what looked like milk and going up through my nostril. I had to be attached to this all day, so I couldn't leave my room. They also had to flush this tube out every day which was a bit uncomfortable.

The third day was tough, trying to communicate with people seemed impossible and I couldn't see it improving. While in hospital, I saw a speech therapist, a dietitian and a physiotherapist and they were all lovely and a great support. The nurses deal with it every day and are marvellous. I was discharged after a week and was delighted.

My next appointment was in one week, to get stitches removed, get the results on the section they had taken away, and also to see what the next step was. At my next appointment they brought me in and explained that the tumour was larger than they thought, and they would have to do the neck dissection to remove lymph nodes in case the cancer had spread. This was Wednesday. They booked me in for the Thursday, to be done on Friday. I was placed on the Max-Fax ward again for the same procedure as before. I was brought to the surgical ward, then to the anaesthetic ward, then into theatre. The consultant popped in again to say hi and to see how I was feeling.

I woke up in recovery. I was very comfortable and after a while I was brought back to the ward. I wasn't allowed sit up or move as I had drain tubes attached to my neck, and I was also attached to a drip.

Next day the nurse helped me to get washed and changed. I felt so much better for it even though it took all my energy. The drains were attached to two small bags which were uncomfortable and awkward, but the nurse gave me a pillowcase to put them in which was easier and meant I didn't need to look at them.

I also didn't look at or touch my scar for the first day. The second day I plucked up the courage to look and try to clean the area. I looked like Frankenstein but it was okay; the drains made it look a lot worse.

The third day was really difficult. I was so tired and I couldn't see my neck improving; also the bruising looked bad.

Every day they checked the drains to see if the fluids had reduced. I was allowed to leave after a week, but I had to return to get the staples out. I didn't come back up. I got them out in my doctor's surgery, because it was over an hour's drive to the hospital.

Having the staples removed made a huge difference. I felt that the neck dissection was a lot worse to recover from than the tongue, physically and emotionally. You can't see the tongue, but the neck is 'in your face', literally; it's what people see first. Also the pain and side effects were worse after the neck surgery. I had neck pain, shoulder pain, an electric-shock-type pain in my tongue and neck, and numbness in my neck, cheek and tongue.

After everything settled down I started physiotherapy for my arm as I had lost the strength in it. With this sort of surgery I think you need to take a step back and let yourself recover. It may not look like a lot of surgery but I feel it really affects your body and you need to take your recovery step by step.

Challenges

I suffer with extreme tiredness. My speech can be slurred when I'm tired. I get frustrated when I can't get some words out. I don't like my husband touching that side of my neck. Only sometimes does my scar bother me; every once in a while I get upset because of it.

Suggestions

> ➤ When having a meal, make sure you're comfortable and relaxed. It's very hard at the beginning to eat if there is a lot going on around you. Give yourself lots of time and plenty to drink

> ➤ Cut food into smaller pieces and chew with your mouth open until you get used to your circumstances and the feeling or numbness in your mouth. On a few occasions I forgot that I couldn't do what I had done before

Conclusion

I think I'm extremely lucky. I have four children, a great husband and a brilliant family. They helped me all the way. Also, because they caught it early, my treatment wasn't as severe as it might have been.

———— ◆ ————

EH

PRIOR TO DIAGNOSIS I WAS leading a hectic life. We had just moved into our newly renovated house, I had a six-month-old baby, a seven year old and a three year old as well. My plan was to return to work full-time a month later. When I first visited my GP with a lump on my neck I was surprised when she suggested further investigations and a visit to a consultant ENT. I was too busy for CT scans and biopsies and I thought it was all an overreaction to an enlarged lymph node. I was well, had no signs of ill health or disease. I knew my body and I felt I was fit and well!

I was very wrong. From my day of diagnosis I lost all confidence in my intuition. I no longer knew my body and every ache and pain would be greeted with mistrust and uncertainty. I had this swollen gland on my neck for maybe six weeks prior to seeking medical intervention. I was so pompous in my attitude that I had discounted it as an after-effect of a cold. I am a nurse and I have nursed people with head and neck cancer. I never put myself in the same category. I was female, 40 years old, had never smoked and rarely drank. The small white spots on my tongue which looked like thrush caused me no pain or discomfort.

Once I was diagnosed I was so amazed that there was a whole set of professionals ready to start working with me to treat and rehabilitate me. A plan was set in motion and my journey started. The overall reaction of people and family was one of shock! Most people automatically think of breast cancer in the under forties.

Challenges

I was fortunate to have my surgery and chemotherapy in the Mater Hospital. My radiotherapy was in the Mater Private. At times a bed was unavailable for chemotherapy, and this caused me huge anxiety. My fear on leaving hospital was that if I became unwell I wouldn't get back in and I'd be left in A&E. This fear was realised one weekend when I was unwell and needed admission. No bed was available, so I left against medical advice. I was later admitted and required three weeks of treatment for radiotoxicity.

There have been many challenges, from neck stiffness to dry mouth. Some have resolved over time, some remain and are my constant reminder. My greatest challenge during treatment was poor appetite and sore mouth. A PEG tube and pain medication helped a lot.

A side effect of the medication was that I felt numb and emotionless, but perhaps that was also my coping mechanism. Finance was also an issue.

I was given immense support and advice from the social work department in the Mater and the head and neck nurse. I cannot praise the head and neck nurse enough. She was, and still is, fantastic. She was the first person I saw after my diagnosis and she managed to convey information in a very relaxed and supportive manner. Her air of confidence gave me and my family huge belief and optimism that I would beat this cancer.

Solutions

Take it one day at a time! Or sometimes one hour at a time.

Resources

Initially I was looking on the internet but I found it too overwhelming as only the bad cases and situations are documented, especially on forums.

The Dublin Dental Hospital information book was good, along with the cancer care book and treatment pack from the oncology nurse.

The speech therapist and dietitian had a huge input in my case.

Food and diet

Yoghurts and soup featured a lot in my diet during treatment and rehabilitation.

Buy good quality products – you deserve the best. Cully & Sully soup and Marks & Spencer creamy yoghurts are great. I ate Chinese chicken and sweetcorn soup direct from the carry-out, and I always had Heinz Farley's Rusks (some people may prefer Liga) to hand – I like mine with hot milk. It was real comfort food.

I love Jamie Oliver's macaroni cheese recipe. It's easy to make, it's not an excessively strong flavour to tolerate and it's easy-peasy to eat.

At night I still enjoy a cup of hot milk with rich tea biscuits dipped in.

Stews and casseroles still feature in my daily menu. I have to have moist food, with sauces or gravy, at all times. Porridge, cereal with hot milk, tea, coffee (although these do reduce saliva), water, custard, bananas, rice pudding, sponge cakes (depending on how crumbly it is) are all good.

I have good and bad days with my appetite. Eating can become tiresome at times. I have become better at eating out and in front of people, but it still is a problem at times. I have become better at knowing my limitations. Foods such as steak, bread rolls and fried chicken are a thing of the past. I still find myself trying to talk while eating, but it's a disaster.

Anything spicy or salty I have to avoid. I also avoid tomato-based dishes, sausages, ketchup, icing on cakes, chocolate, alcohol of any kind, fizzy drinks, citrus juices, crisps, popcorn, sweets, crackers, some fruits (grapes, apples, oranges) and extremes of hot and cold.

Life today

My speech is improving. I find the clarity of my speech varies depending on my degree of tiredness and the time of day.

I still have saliva but not as much. I drink water throughout the day. I always have water to hand. A dry mouth definitely affects my speech, too much and my speech is wet. I have a daily dental regime. I have to maintain my dental hygiene to avoid decay.

Fatigue has always been my greatest battle. When I feel well I am busy and probably exhaust myself and need to go to bed. My diet has an impact on this. I am still trying to work on this and eat regularly. My lack of appetite sometimes enables me to go many hours without eating.

Conclusion

I would love to have a social network of people who have had head and neck cancer; there's very limited support. I feel that people don't appreciate the after-effects of this cancer and how it has impacted my life.

Joseph Furlong

I WAS FIRST DIAGNOSED WITH a carcinoma of the tongue in 1999. At that time I was a patient in Our Lady of Lourdes Hospital in Drogheda, where I was getting treatment for a disc problem. I had what I thought was a blister on my tongue for about six months at this time, which was causing me only slight discomfort. At no time was I in pain.

I had a biopsy done in hospital and I was told it was cancer. I had never heard of head and neck cancer before this. I have to say that I was a very heavy smoker – two to three packs per day – so I wasn't really surprised.

I was sent to St James's Hospital in January 2000 and I was told surgery was the best option. The treatment and pain control I received in St James's Hospital was second to none. Although I was advised all the way through the procedure as to what was happening, I think more should be done after the treatment regarding the nerve damage to face and neck.

My eating and speech were affected but I had great help from the speech therapist. For the first month I was on soft food only, chicken and fish and soup. Sometimes swallowing is still a problem. I still get pain in my tongue and neck but it's manageable. Dry mouth is also a problem and I always watch what I am eating. The disfigurement is not an issue for me as I grew a beard to cover the scars.

In 2005 and again in 2009 the cancer returned, again on my tongue and again I had surgery. Each time I recovered more quickly but I was left feeling very anxious, so I asked for and received help in dealing with this.

I feel okay now and I only have myself to blame because I smoked so much. I also consider myself very lucky as my cancer could have been somewhere else in my body and a lot worse.

I am receiving ongoing treatment at the Dental Hospital and have monthly check-ups at St James's Hospital.

Suggestions

The after-effects of the operation should be better explained so that you know what's normal or not. I found my second time in Intensive Care to be horrible. The nurse didn't understand what I was saying, and trying to explain I wanted a bed-pan, until it was too late, was very degrading. It put me off the ICU for life.

Anne L'Hénoret

I WAS DIAGNOSED IN MARCH 2010 with cancer of the tongue. My only symptoms were that for about four weeks I had felt like I was getting a sore throat when I first woke up in the mornings. A little tickle, that's all. Usually, as soon as I had water or coffee it would disappear. So it was barely a conscious thing, as it was a very mild sensation at a time of day when I was just about awake.

The only reason I found out what it really was, was that one weekend I was going away to London and I had a sore tooth, so I used Listerine to avoid getting an infection while I was abroad (I normally didn't use mouthwash). Each time I used it I got that sensation again, this time much more noticeably, as it happened several times a day (the alcohol in Listerine was stinging, basically).

So I had a look in my throat and discovered a hole in the left side of my tongue, right at the back near the root. I could fit the end of a finger into it. I asked my husband to take a photo of it, as it was hard for me to see in the mirror. When I saw it I had an idea that it could be cancerous. I have an interest in anatomy and health matters from my training as a yoga teacher and holistic therapist, so this is why I had some idea it could be a carcinoma. I was not aware of head and neck cancers as such but I knew carcinomas can affect soft tissue anywhere in the body.

I e-mailed the photo to a friend who is a dentist that night as I wasn't sure if this was something a dentist or a GP would deal with. She said anything in the mouth is for the dentist to deal with so I went to see her as soon as possible. She and her colleague thought it very unlikely to be cancer as I didn't fit the profile. I had given up smoking ten years previously, I drank very little, ate well, I was fit and young (36 years old) and I was working as a yoga teacher and charity worker. I had never been sick before. But I had not cut myself with my toothbrush or had any other trauma that I could recall, so to make sure, they referred me to the Dental Hospital to see a soft tissue specialist. I think that was on a Friday.

The minute the consultant saw the sore she requested a biopsy and told me it would be fast-tracked from three weeks to three days and that I would know on the following Tuesday. She didn't say it was definitely cancer but obviously, the way she was handling it, it was clear she thought it probably was. She did say that if it was cancer, it had been caught quite early so we could deal with it. On the Tuesday morning, first thing, it was confirmed.

I feel I was lucky to have had such a prompt diagnosis, thanks to a quick referral to the right place. I am quite an anxious person in times of uncertainty. I deal with difficulties well, usually, and I don't mind hard work if I am very clear on what needs to be done. You could say I am rather 'black and white'. So for me it would have been very stressful to go from doctor to doctor for ages trying to find answers, which can happen, especially if the cancer is internal. At least with the mouth it is easy to see and to do a biopsy.

To add to my luck the surgeon who would operate on me was in the Dental Hopsital that Tuesday, so I was introduced to him immediately and again by chance his clinic is on a Wednesday every week. That day the PET scan and other tests were arranged, bloods and X-rays taken etc. All this was to determine how advanced the cancer was, if it was in the lymph etc. The surgeon was very positive and extremely straightforward which I was glad of. I didn't want any shilly-shallying, and I really trusted him from day one, which I think is hugely important. He asked if I had questions or concerns and I told him my work involves talking all the time – I teach for a living – and he said, 'I have never shut anyone up yet.' So we started off with both confidence and humour.

I think the rest of the tests must have taken two to three weeks. I don't quite remember; it was all a whirlwind really. I remember that Easter meant some delays in getting test results back but it was still pretty fast and efficient. Eventually I had an assessment of how advanced it was, the cancer was not present in the lymph but it was relatively big for such an awkward place at the root of the tongue, which affects speaking and eating.

I remember it being a very busy time, which was just as well, as it left me less time to think: there were lots of medical appointments, I told my friends and family and my students, I organised handover of my yoga classes. In some ways I was on a kind of high. There was a sense of being pulled out of normality, of having this big job to do, almost an 'adventure'. So for me that was not a particularly difficult time, as it sort of took me out of myself. One particularly rough moment though was telling my best friend. She lost her sister to cancer at the same age. That was horrible; she was so upset, and I knew she would be, but she was an absolute rock throughout the experience.

Of course the truth is that I had no idea really of what was going to happen and I am sure I would have struggled a lot more with the plan, had I really known what was to come!

Practicalities

For me the treatment was tough in many ways, like for everyone. But I had a couple of advantages in that I didn't live too far away from the hospitals and I had great support from family and friends. Also I was very fit when it happened so I tried to go for treatment under my own steam when I could, I cycled six miles to radiotherapy for the first few weeks before I became too tired. With head and neck cancers it is possible to still be very active, as the rest of the body can move normally. It helped me stay in shape, but most of all it was a big thing for me mentally to not feel like a cancer patient all the time.

Cancer: the word and what it means

I feel strongly that the word *cancer* is very misleading or inaccurate, in a sense, as it covers such a huge range of problems and experiences. Also many of the problems we experience stem in fact from the treatment and that again varies hugely.

I had very serious surgery, lost part of my tongue, had my lip and jaw cut in half, and a neck dissection which permanently affects the neck and shoulder muscles, fascia and nerves. I had to learn to eat and speak all over again and I had six weeks of radiotherapy which caused a lot of fatigue and dry mouth, and for three months I lost my sense of taste. But the rest of me was well, and I didn't have chemotherapy, which sounds really tough, so my experience was totally different from someone else with cancer. That's one of the things I feel about that word *cancer*.

The word *cancer* can also mark you as a patient or a victim, and can almost erase the rest of your personality. To other people you can become 'that person who is dealing with cancer' and, afterwards, a 'cancer survivor'. I wasn't going to go down that road. Yes I was dealing with all this and it was pretty all encompassing for a good six months, but I was still me, not just a cancer patient.

Also, many people talk about it as a battle. I can see why and I am sure it is really helpful to think that way – it is definitely better than feeling pessimistic about the outcome – but for me it sounds a bit odd, because I don't feel anyone attacked me. I don't like the war terminology. It is just something that happened. Life is random. Of course we can help the odds with our lifestyle etc, but still it is too simplistic to say we get cancer because we are victims of something. I also didn't have that question many people seem to ask themselves, *Why me? Why did it happen to me? Did I do something wrong?* To me, it doesn't work like that.

Low points

Of course I got angry and frustrated sometimes with the pain, with what felt like lack of progress, sometimes with the rehabilitation exercises and especially with the fatigue.

But for me there were two low points in the treatment. There was the day, about seven or eight days after surgery, when I was allowed to try drinking water (I had been fed by tube for days) and I couldn't even keep it in my mouth, never mind swallow it. It was a Friday and they said, 'Keep trying; see you on Monday.'

It was terrifying because at the weekends I didn't see the speech therapist, who was helping me with swallowing again, and so for those very, very long days I thought I would never drink or eat again and I'd be fed by tube for ever. It turned out it was just going to take time and a lot of hard work. Swallowing is learned as a baby and we have no conscious sense of it, so when it doesn't work and we have to learn it again, it is very strange and difficult.

I would say to anyone going through swallow and speech therapy: don't be discouraged. It takes time and it is sore and tedious, but it works. It's the same with physiotherapy, if your neck is affected for example.

I recovered everything eventually. I don't have pain, I can move normally, I can eat everything I want and I speak all day in my job. I know I had amazing luck in how well I recovered, and I owe it to the amazing therapists I had, but I also owe it to myself.

I worked very hard at it and I really want other people in the situation to know that it is worth doing the painful boring exercises every day, even if you are tired. They work! I had a head start as a yoga teacher. Because I believed in stretching and repeating exercises anyway, I started stretching when I was still in hospital, but I have to say, the teams make it very easy to do the right things. You don't need to understand how it works for it to give results. Just do it, do as they say.

The other big problem was fatigue later on, post-radiotherapy. More on that below.

Fear

Weirdly, I never thought I could die from this; it never even occurred to me. I didn't become afraid of this thing until around 18 to 24 months after the treatment. At that point, sometimes, going to check-ups I would get very scared or in the middle of the night I'd get scared. My life was totally back to normal and I hardly ever thought about it. No one ever mentioned it around me anymore, and then it would creep up on me, this fear: could it be back and I don't know? Can I really let my guard down? Am I checking often enough?

The psychologists call it hyper-vigilance or Damocles syndrome. It is normal, especially if, like me, you found the cancer yourself. Was it really 'that easy'? I know it sounds weird, it wasn't easy at all, but it was dealt with. I recovered really well, everything is normal bar a few scars and an unusual way of eating and talking (which other people don't notice and has become normal to me). OK, I am very thirsty when I wake up, but I am used to that too. Is that it? It can't be …

It is a weird emotional rollercoaster, being so grateful that everything is normal and being afraid that it could be taken away again at the next check-up, because I know my tongue now isn't really big enough for any more to be cut off and still be able to talk and eat well. I can't have radiotherapy again in the same site, so if it comes back I am looking at a very bleak picture.

I know how close I came to living a very different life, being fed through a tube and not being understood when I speak, so I sometimes get really scared of that happening. It is a visceral terror, actually, but thankfully I don't feel it very often.

I think when the medical appointments become less frequent, there's another opportunity for the fear to come, as there is no longer constant reassurance. At three years post-treatment, I feel more relaxed again.

Fatigue

Fatigue was a big problem for me for ages. Radiotherapy didn't seem to affect me too badly at the time, but for so long after I had this weird, really annoying, tiredness. I like a busy life – work, socialising, sport, and I drive myself quite hard too in that I want to do things to a high standard.

At its worst the fatigue made my body feel like a stone and my mind numb. The physical fatigue didn't last as long as the mental, gradually improving over a period of about a year, and I was able to get rid of the physical fatigue by moving about and not resting too much.

I would advise forcing yourself to do a bit of exercise, or a lot, depending on your previous fitness level, as it takes you out of the feeling of tiredness. It is a balancing act: sometimes you must give in to the fatigue and rest, but don't do it all the time or you'll feel worse. Make yourself do things and socialise, too. Resting too much made me feel depressed, whereas distractions and activity definitely helped me to feel better.

While you are very tired, e.g. during or soon after treatment, a good DVD box set is great. During radiotherapy and the weeks immediately after, I had everyone lend me some of those. After coming home from radiotherapy every day, I had a routine. I wouldn't nap as such (I couldn't sleep during the day) but I'd watch one or two episodes of something instead, to rest.

The mental fatigue, however, I struggled with enormously, and I still do. I do not have the mental agility I had before and it really frustrates me. I forget things, I feel my mind is often blank. It has improved over time, and again it is better if I force myself, but my mind does not seem to respond to retraining the same way my body did.

People tell me it is aging, but at 39 I am not accepting that! Or it is because of my busy new job, but it doesn't feel like me. It is a different sort of fatigue; it isn't like being tired from doing lots of stuff. Sleep doesn't always relieve it, and it's a feeling that is very hard to describe to others. I feel a bit like I am pinned to a bed or sofa and staring at nothing. To be fair it does get better with time, but at one point it felt like it would never stop dominating my life and I had to really practise accepting this kind of 'slowing down'. Accepting but not giving in to it, that's the trick.

Appearance

For me, this has not been too big an issue. My surgeon did an amazing job so my scar, while very long (all down my neck and across my chin and lip), is really very discreet, considering. I used Dermatix gel to help heal it and some gentle self-massage, both of which have really helped.

It took some getting used to, especially for my husband of course, but most people don't really notice. I do have a bit of sagging and a few new wrinkles around the mouth, so on a bad day if I look in the mirror when I am tired I might feel a bit prematurely aged, but it rarely bothers me. I am alive and eating and talking and I am so grateful for that. The functionality is so much more important that the scar. And on other days I even think it is kind of cool, actually. After all the treatment was finished I went and totally changed my hairstyle, so I look really different anyway and people notice that, not the scar!

—— ♦ ——

CANCER OF THE SUB-MANDIBULAR GLAND

JK

I WAS SITTING AROUND ON my own overthinking, so I rang my sister. She knew I had been for a biopsy the previous week on the lump I had first noticed under my left jawline two months previously. It was only day six and I had been informed in St James's Hospital that it would take at least a week for the results to reach my consultant. However, my anxiety was rising and we decided I should make a call. The consultant's secretary told me she would follow up on my query in relation to when the biopsy result would come through. She rang me back within half an hour and said the results were being faxed over. Could I come in for a very early appointment the next morning? I knew at that moment that the tumour was malignant and I had cancer.

This was late November 2008. Just to give a little background to my life at the time: I was and still am living in Glenageary, County Dublin. I am married and my husband and I have three children who were then aged two, six and nine. I had worked as a secondary school teacher but was lucky enough to be able to take time out to stay at home with my children in their early years. All in all a pretty normal existence.

In late September I noticed a small, almond-shaped lump under my jaw when I was putting on make-up. I had undergone a routine annual check-up a few weeks earlier with my doctor and all blood tests etc. had come back clear, so I didn't get overly stressed about it. When the lump didn't disappear and seemed to be growing larger, I rang and made an appointment to see the GP in late October. At this visit, following an examination, the doctor said the main possibility was that this was a blocked salivary (submandibular) gland and he was going to refer me to a consultant for further investigation.

When I received my appointment date it was four weeks away. This troubled me a bit, as when I did my own research (Google!) into the symptoms of a blocked salivary gland I found out that it was supposed to be painful and I was not experiencing any discomfort at all. However, anything more ominous, like a tumour, seemed to be exceptionally rare so I decided not to overreact. Also the doctor seemed to have a lot of faith in the consultant he was referring me to so I decided I would like to be in a good pair of hands. I would hold out.

This consultant was the first in a long line of excellent and compassionate medical professionals that I met on my cancer journey. He refrained from using the word *cancer,* instead discussing 'cells that had to be dealt with', while reminding me of the huge leaps and bounds that have been made in cancer treatment. My husband and I left his office (after tea for the shock) with a referral to see a surgeon. The next few days were a haze of shock and adrenaline. We filtered out the information to family and close friends while trying to keep some level of normality for the children who were oblivious to it all.

Within days I met with the ENT consultant at his office in the Blackrock Clinic. He assessed the situation, telling me that he would like to complete the surgery to remove the tumour this side of Christmas. I was happy with that. I just wanted it out as soon as possible. While I waited for the date for surgery I did the Christmas Santa toy shopping for the children and prayed I would get to do it many more times in the future.

Things began to move very quickly. I got a bed in the Eye and Ear Hospital in Dublin for 6 December, with surgery booked for 8 December. Prior to surgery I had a series of CAT scans in St Vincent's Hospital. My sister, who worked nearby, kept a near constant vigil and played a big part in keeping me from contemplating worst possible scenarios. Other amazing family and friends helped my husband keep things afloat at home.

Prior to surgery I was told about the possible complications of the operation. Because of the proximity of the tumour to facial nerves there was a very real possibility that these could be damaged, depending on what needed to be done during the surgery. If this happened it would lead to some kind of facial paralysis on the left side of my face. I accepted this risk without question. I didn't think my kids would care what I looked like as long as I was around.

In my hazy memory I think surgery took about three to three and a half hours. On waking, I was told that everything had gone very well and that they hadn't needed to remove the parotid gland (the salivary gland near the ear and close to the submandibular gland). They removed the submandibular gland and tumour and a large number of lymph nodes surrounding it. It was a relief to have the surgery over.

This sense of relief was tempered a few days later when I was told a small shadow had been noted on my liver during one of my previous scans in St Vincent's. In fairness I was told that this was not necessarily a sign of something ominous as sometimes women of my age can get a cyst on the liver. Once again my practical sister had to remind me that you can only deal with the information you are given. This was hard advice to follow but probably the best piece of advice that I got through my illness.

A few days after surgery I had a visit from the ENT consultant who told me the results of the tests on the tumour. It was an aggressive and very rare type called a carcinosarcoma. Later, questioning my consultants about this type of cancer, they informed me there is no known cause for this type of cancer except a very small link to radiation exposure in the workplace (of which I have had none). The consultant said I would require radiotherapy but the main positive news was that, as far as could be ascertained, the margins were clear. This meant that no identifiable spread had occurred.

He told me not to worry about the liver scan. He was sure it would be fine. A few hours later the radiographer in St Vincent's said he was right; it was just a cyst. The relief was overwhelming and I felt I had just taken a few steps back from the edge of a precipice.

I was delighted to get home after eight days in hospital. Christmas passed and the large scar healed up. The left side of my face, while numb, seemed to be fine, with no discernible damage thanks to the skilled hands of the consultant.

In January I made my first trip to St Luke's Hospital in Rathgar to visit Professor Donal Hollywood and his team to discuss my radiotherapy treatment. It is poignant to be writing about this at this time, as Professor Hollywood passed away so recently. I consider myself so privileged to have been under his excellent care for the last four and a half years. On my first visit Professor Hollywood, in a gentle way, strongly recommended I have radiotherapy treatment to minimise any possibility of a recurrence of the cancer. Radiotherapy is the accepted gold-standard treatment for this type of cancer. I was fine with this suggestion.

I had experience of a family member going through radiotherapy and I knew the routine. Or so I thought! I was given an appointment to see a consultant dentist in the Dublin Dental Hospital. As the radiotherapy would be hitting my jaw this could cause issues with my teeth and any compromised teeth would have to be removed. I didn't take this too seriously as I felt my teeth were in good condition and all would be well.

The visit to the Dublin Dental Hospital brought me into contact with a wonderful consultant, who would oversee my care. Following X-rays, despite my teeth being in relatively good condition, it was decided that I would have to have three teeth removed from the bottom row, one of which had been recently crowned (all that money!) and two of which were filled teeth. Also, a tooth at the back of my upper jaw was grinding on the inside of my cheek and causing damage, which might be aggravated during treatment. So four teeth in total.

This, for some reason, was a very low moment. I just was not expecting this sideswipe. I was feeling a bit battle-weary, and for two minutes I thought about walking out and taking my chances that surgery alone would be enough. But how would I explain that one to my kids if it came back? Needless to say the teeth were removed under sedation and the gums were allowed to heal for a few weeks.

After that there were still two more procedures to complete. First I had to get a mould made of my teeth in order to create two trays to fit onto my upper and lower teeth. Following radiotherapy I would have to use these trays on my teeth for 15 minutes a night. The trays would contain prescribed solutions that would both keep my teeth strong and prevent decay. Because radiotherapy treatment weakens the jawbone, any infection or decay could cause major difficulty. The trays are part of the 'prevention is better than a cure' approach, to ensure no decay sets in.

The second procedure was to get a stent made to keep my tongue out of the way during radiotherapy so it would not be caught in the crossfire and damaged. Another consultant made this piece of equipment, which was at best uncomfortable, but I understood the necessity of it.

Back in St Luke's, I was fitted for a thermoplastic mask to prevent movement of my head and shoulders during treatment. The nurses gave me advice on what to expect in terms of side effects. I was told there may be difficulty eating due to dry mouth, mouth ulcers, lack of taste etc. They also discussed skin damage and a sunburn effect, which they recommended treating with E45 cream. In the end I didn't have as many side effects as I had anticipated. It takes a lot to put me off my food!

When it came to doing a dummy run of a radiotherapy session with my tongue stent in place and the mask on, I assumed I would be fine. This was not the case. I hit a big wall. I felt claustrophobic and panicky. I asked the radiation therapists what the procedure was if I couldn't last the few minutes required. They said it was possible to do it under sedation as then I would be fully relaxed. I didn't want to go for this option as I was planning to drive to and from St Luke's for the sessions, of which there would be 33 in total.

Returning home, I did some sessions on relaxation with a trained psychotherapist. Sometimes I practised at home with the stent in my mouth to try to overcome the negative sensation of it. I did this while listening to music, which I intended to bring with me to radiotherapy sessions as this was accommodated in the hospital. This made me feel much more in control.

Eventually the treatment got underway. I stuck on the CD of Tibetan chants and told myself I could do it for the few minutes I had to. I put in the stent and hopped on the table. The lights went down. I listened to the music while I imagined I was following someone (no idea who!) up a grassy mountain that looked like the Alps in the summer, and I let myself breathe. If I couldn't cope the radiotherapists told me to raise my hand and they would be right in. I didn't have to raise my hand. I was proud of myself that day. I felt I had taken control of the situation, and that cancer had not managed to make me a victim.

The weeks passed by quickly – February, March and finally into April. My husband or I, or friends of ours, dropped the children to school. Work was still going on for my husband and we asked a girl to come in for a few hours to help me three days a week in the afternoon. My appointment was usually at 10.30 a.m. While in St Luke's I was constantly buoyed up by how attentive the staff were and what a good atmosphere prevailed at the heart of the hospital. While there I was offered counselling sessions. I availed of two sessions and had a good rant about feelings I didn't want to distress my family with. They also encouraged me to have reflexology on site, which I did a few times.

The people who were having treatment alongside me were inspirational and I enjoyed talking to them. I vowed I would try not to moan too much when I would catch a glimpse of a child being wheeled around the hospital. That's when cancer really isn't fair at all. As I said, I didn't experience many side effects. I didn't lose much weight and although my face and neck did burn a bit, they were easily soothed. Professor Hollywood also monitored me throughout this time.

On the last day of radiotherapy the nurses offered me the mask I wore to bring home. I was bemused by this as I could not wait to see the back of it. Some people, the radiotherapists said, bring it home and make something artistic out of it or grow flowers up through it in the garden. I didn't take it home. I kind of regret that now. It would have made a great dartboard!

The five months between diagnosis and finishing treatment are hard to describe in terms of the emotional impact. I experienced every possible feeling from despair to elation. My system felt like it was continually in fight-or-flight mode. In the worst moments, I was deeply worried that my children could potentially be without a mother and my husband would be left to bring them up on his own, which would be difficult, brilliant as he is. It took a while for this fear to recede and that is probably quite normal.

In the throes of treatment I thought I would never feel carefree again. Four years later, with each check-up that goes by, I realise that this is not the case. There is also an interesting expectation out there that if someone has faced a serious illness, they will be motivated to transform their lives into something beyond amazing. While this would be wonderful it is not always realistic. Any dreams I may harbour to backpack around the world will have to come after the usual midlife stuff of bringing up kids and working part-time. I am just glad I am here to do that, and I do try harder to see the beauty in an ordinary day.

Four months after treatment finished I started a part-time job lecturing. After eight years of working at home this was another challenge I found scary, but in a positive way. It certainly gave me something to focus on other than cancer. I also took up running, from which I get a sense of well-being and achievement, though 10 km is my limit!

I still let the small stuff get to me sometimes, which I know I shouldn't do, so my next plan is to take up yoga. I am hoping this will give me the demeanour of the Dalai Lama!

I never really forget completely that I've had cancer. However, I can do a pretty impressive job of ignoring it on a day-to-day basis, except for check-up days. I have six-monthly check-ups that alternate between my surgeon and my oncologist. These can involve a scope examination or the occasional chest X-ray. I also have a yearly dental check-up in the Dublin Dental Hospital, and I still have to use the trays on my teeth most nights. This is a pain, but it seems to be maintaining my teeth, so it is worth it.

I make sure not to miss my appointments, as I know how lucky I am to have access to a health system that is monitoring me so well. In conclusion I want to pay tribute to all the medical staff I encountered along the way. I could not have been in more professional and caring hands and I am grateful to every one of them.

If you are reading this and are in a similar situation, I hope all goes well for you. And watch out for that light at the end of the tunnel – it gets bigger with every step forward.

CANCER OF THE TONSIL

GP

My year-long experience with cancer, as a 33-year-old Irish female

I STILL FIND IT HARD to believe that it happened to me. When I look back at 2012, it appears like a movie in my mind's eye, though surely not of my life but someone else's?

But it was me.

I had just returned from my first trip to Paris with friends over the bank holiday weekend in October 2011. I can't remember the exact timing, whether it was morning or night, but I do remember I was carrying out my daily skincare routine when I felt a small swelling on the left hand side of my throat, quite close to my jawline. I thought nothing of it. I am the type of person who gets every cold and flu going during winter, so my first thought was that I was getting a sore throat. And that was it.

It was five weeks later on a Monday morning in work when I started to feel slightly anxious about the swelling. I suspected it was getting bigger. I asked one of my colleagues to accompany me to the bathroom; she looked bemused by my request. I pointed to my neck and asked her to tell me if she could see a swelling or was it my imagination. She confirmed that it did indeed exist and suggested that I visit my GP. But she assured me it was likely something that may have to be drained and nothing more. She was older and therefore wiser than me, so I didn't even question this explanation.

That same day, I was in my GP's office apologising for being a hypochondriac. But she went ahead and took blood and told me not to worry. Two days later the tests had come back clear and I was told that as my white blood cell count was perfectly normal there was nothing sinister about the swelling. I was given a week's supply of antibiotics and told to check in the following week. But the swelling was still there a week later, and it felt quite tender at this stage. My GP suggested it could be an issue with my teeth so I made an appointment for 16 December 2011 with my new dentist.

My dentist sent me for X-rays in the Charlemont Clinic but they provided no answers in relation to the swelling. Thankfully, for me, my dentist was concerned enough to suggest that I see a consultant. With letters from both my GP and dentist I got an appointment for an ENT clinic in St James's Hospital.

It was strange that despite being a computer-dependent individual I didn't even google the consultant to see what kind of work he specialises in. If I had, I may have been more prepared for the outcome. But, finding myself newly single in 2011 after seven years, I was heading off to Barcelona for New Year's Eve, and I didn't give my appointment a second thought.

I had high hopes for 2012 as I was starting a new job that I was really excited about. On Friday 20 January I went to see the ENT consultant, mortified that I had to ask for a half-day in my first week.

I was so naive, I didn't even contemplate it being anything serious. To me it was just an inconvenience, something I wanted fixed without any further hassle. Even as I sat in the waiting room with patients who were physically disfigured, I still hadn't even checked to see what kind of specialist I was seeing. Maybe I knew on some level, but nothing registered in my brain.

Luckily my parents had insisted on coming with me that day.

My first shock was the scope. The doctor inserted a camera up my nose and down my throat to look at the swelling. I had never been in hospital prior to this day except as a child of maybe five or six, so even this procedure threw me.

The second shock was the biopsy, even just hearing a doctor speak those words to you is surreal. I suppose I had always imagined a biopsy to be like taking blood, but it was actually quite painful. I was told the results would take about three weeks. I left the hospital feeling sore and anxious. My parents' worried faces only served to highlight the gravity of the situation.

But still I didn't really comprehend what was going on. I spent the next week totally focused on my job. But the following Thursday I saw three missed calls from the hospital. A doctor asked that I come into the clinic the next day as my results were back. I remember thinking how efficient they were. I thought it would take three weeks. Again, it didn't even register that this was a bad sign. Although I complained about the fact that I had meetings to attend, the doctor quietly assured me that I really needed to see him.

My mother insisted on coming into the doctor's room with me this time. My sister works in healthcare and had told my parents it could be bad news, but no one told me.

When the doctor started to tell me that the biopsy had proved positive for cancerous cells, I just couldn't take it in. I was staring at my mother's heartbroken face, willing myself to listen to the doctor's words. But it was like I was under water; I could hear sound but no actual words. I asked my mother to leave the room as I couldn't take the look on her face. The doctor said I needed to go in for surgery straight away, that it was urgent. I wanted to throw up.

I spent the next three days ringing St James's Hospital daily at 11 a.m. and 2 p.m., trying to get a bed. I hadn't realised that you had to wait for a bed when a doctor tells you your surgery is urgent; it didn't make sense to me. I thought I could drop dead at any moment. Finally, the doctor booked me in for the PET scan so that I would at least be in the hospital. Whilst I was getting the scan, my father went to Admissions; he broke down in tears in front of them and I was offered a bed that evening. I'm not sure if the tears were the persuading factor or if it was just good timing. My mother referred to that doctor as a saint from that day on.

The surgery was a success; they removed the tumour from my neck and a number of lymph nodes. As they were still not sure where the primary source of the cancer was, they also took a number of biopsies from the mouth and throat area.

Two weeks after I had been discharged from hospital, I went back into the ENT clinic for the biopsy results. I had actually convinced myself at this stage that they had got it wrong, that it wasn't actually cancer. Originally, they had thought it was in my parotid gland but when they performed the surgery they found that it wasn't this gland at all which basically means that my scar is not as big as I had prepared myself for. So I thought that if they could get that wrong, maybe the diagnosis was wrong too.

But it was confirmed on that visit in February that I had grade 3 tonsillar cancer. Fortunately, the surgeons had taken the precaution of removing my tonsils, so I did not need another operation. But sitting in that chair with my mother by my side, being told I would need the full course of radiation and also chemotherapy, I felt like the rug had been ripped out from beneath my feet. I just couldn't believe it. I was young, I ate healthily, I exercised regularly, I was a size 10 – how the hell could this happen to me?

It's funny how the brain works when you're in shock. Yes, I had tears in my eyes as the doctor explained the treatment I would need, but all I could think about at that moment was whether he was single!

The next few months were a mixture of emotions: anger, denial, despair, confusion. And I wasn't the only one feeling like that; my parents and sisters were devastated. My friends were at a loss.

Again, I was dumbfounded at the process. I would never have guessed how long you have to wait to start treatment. I was fully diagnosed in early February 2012, yet I didn't actually start treatment until late April. There were a number of reasons. First, I suffered complications after my first surgery and had to have an emergency surgery two weeks later, so I needed time for my body to recover from the blood loss.

Another major setback came from a very unlikely place: my teeth. When I was told by St Luke's Hospital (where I was to receive the radiation and chemotherapy) that I would need to go for a check-up in the Dental Hospital in Dublin I didn't give it much thought. They told me that as I was to receive radiation to the lower part of my face, jawline and neck, they needed to check that my teeth were healthy. Well I had been to the dentist a few months prior to this so I just assumed that all would be fine. But what I didn't realise at this stage was that once you have received radiation to this area you cannot have any major dental work done in the future. This is because the irradiated jawbone is permanently at risk of osteoradionecrosis (ORN), which is a non-healing infection of the bone caused by trauma. This means that the dental consultant needs to make a judgement call on what may go wrong with your teeth in the future. I had a number of large fillings and some decay in my back teeth, which under normal circumstances could be easily managed. But with the radiation treatment, this would prove a major issue. I was told I would need five extractions. I was devastated.

I was booked in for dental surgery the following week. I assumed I would be sitting in a dentist's chair for the extractions. I didn't realise I would be under anaesthetic and back in a hospital bed. This being so soon after my other surgeries, I found the whole experience quite traumatic. I was already trying to cope with having a new scar on my neck, and now I would have to deal with bare gums. I felt so unattractive.

After the dental surgery, I was provided with gum trays that I will have to use for the rest of my life to ensure my teeth stay healthy. At first, my nightly teeth regime would take nearly 30 minutes but I have become quite skilled since then and it only takes 15 to 20 minutes now.

A few weeks after the dental surgery I had my first appointment in St Luke's Hospital. Living back home with my parents in Tallaght, I was absolutely delighted to be assigned to St Luke's, as this would mean a very short commute to the hospital. When you are faced with seven weeks of daily radiation and constant nausea, the length of commute is very important.

My treatment plan consisted of daily radiation, Monday to Friday, with five day-long sessions of chemotherapy. The first two weeks were fine. I felt tired but I was in no pain. By week three, nausea became an issue and I started to vomit on a daily basis, and unfortunately this continued for the remaining four weeks of treatment and for three weeks after treatment.

But the team in St Luke's Hospital were just fantastic. It was obviously not pleasant, but I had the full support (and plenty of drugs!) to manage the situation. They literally carry you through the bad times. The head and neck support nurse was like my own personal cheerleader, she was an amazing support to both me and my family.

Due to the location of the cancer, I had great difficulty with eating during treatment. I suffered from dry mouth, so I had to keep a glass of water by my bed at all times. I couldn't eat solid or dry food, instead I depended completely on the build-up drinks and milkshakes recommended by the nutritionist for the duration of my treatment. I struggled to find a drink that didn't make me nauseous. In the end I could only drink the strawberry version. Vanilla ice cream made up the remainder of my diet for those seven weeks.

I finished treatment in June 2012. It took me nearly three months to start eating a varied diet again, and it was even longer until I got my taste buds back.

I lost some hair during treatment, which was another difficult time. The first time I was in the shower and felt something running down my leg. I looked down to see a clump of hair moving towards the drain. I cried for an hour after that. But I was lucky not to lose my full head of hair.

So how do I feel today? Physically I am fine. I got the all-clear in September 2012. (To celebrate I went straight out and bought a red convertible car!) I went back to work in November 2012 on a phased basis as recommended by my team. I felt so grateful that the company I had only worked with for two weeks had kept my job for me. It gave me the motivation and focus I needed to get out there again. It's amazing how quickly you become institutionalised. The fatigue that is associated with treatment can be really frustrating. I want to get back to normal life so badly but I still need to take naps in the afternoon to keep me going. But it is easily managed.

The psychological effect is harder to manage. I was not a very emotional person before this happened to me. Friends and family would often comment on how strong I am, but since the cancer I find myself crying a lot. It left me feeling vulnerable. I felt betrayed by my body. I look in the mirror and don't recognise myself any more. Cancer does change you. I look at the world differently now. I look at my friends and family differently. It gives you clarity on what and who are important in your life.

But I also struggled with finding the positive, and I experienced some very low periods over the past 12 months. I felt there was such pressure to garner the positive from this experience and say that now I would live life to the full, that I learned so much and that it was nearly a blessing in disguise. But most days I just felt anger that I had been robbed of a year of my life. But no matter how angry or depressed I was, I had survived and I was grateful for that. I have been fortunate to have access to a wonderful psychologist in St Luke's Hospital. To be honest I don't know how I would have gotten through this experience without her and I would highly recommend that anyone else going through this find someone that they can talk to because it really does help.

As I write these words, it is a year to the day from my first appointment in St James's Hospital. I am back working three days a week, socialising with friends, hoping to rejoin my running club in a few weeks and looking for a new place to live. I may have been robbed of a year of my life but I am determined that this year will make up for the last.

———◆———

James Lucey

I WAS A 48-YEAR-OLD married father of five, self-employed with no significant medical history apart from gall bladder and appendix issues, albeit that my mother died in 1983 aged 58 with cancer of the colon, and my sister died in 1999 aged 46 with breast cancer. I presented to a locum for my usual GP in July 2005 with a lump on my neck, having become concerned about the lump while shaving. In retrospect I think that the lump may have been developing over a few months. The GP referred me to a consultant ENT specialist at Mallow General Hospital, who in turn referred me to South Infirmary Victoria Hospital (SIVH) Cork. The lump was removed late in August 2005, shortly after the death of my wife's brother, who suffered chronic MS. It was a difficult time for us all.

I didn't have any expectation of malignancy until I was informed by my consultant that the pathology suggested that the tumour that had been removed was a secondary, rather than a primary. He was unclear about what course of action I should now take about the chances of locating the primary cancer. I was left with the impression that the prognosis was very poor.

In somewhat of a panic I contacted a friend who was a medic in Dublin, who arranged for me to be seen by an ENT consultant for a second opinion. He suggested that if my primary was below my clavicle I had little chance of survival but advised that my best chance was the removal of my left tonsil. I had this procedure less than ten days later at SIVH Cork. I attended St Luke's in Rathgar as an outpatient for my radiotherapy and chemotherapy treatments.

Up to this, while I had heard of throat cancer I had no idea that mouth, head and neck cancer was a job lot.

In one way it was paralysing news, but my way of dealing with it was through black humour. My consultant recommended that I recruit someone to replace me in my job. My preparation for the battle ahead now seems like a planned invasion of the medical world, in the sense of not taking no for an answer. This was spearheaded by my wife, who had trained as a nurse and who managed and coordinated everything for me.

I was in a hurry to undergo all the necessary further tests, so much so that my persistence and that of many friends and connections became well known to the secretaries of the medics involved in my treatment. I had little faith in publications on the subject, preferring to discuss the matter directly with the experts, and I found that my many secret forays onto the internet were frightening rather than beneficial. Also, a report on Sky News around the time my treatment started suggested that oral cancer resulted in the main from heavy consumption of alcohol and cigarettes, which was simply not true in my case. I found it offensive.

Our children were at an expensive age. We had three in third level education, one in boarding school and one special needs child at home. Support from family and friends enabled my wife to devote a great deal of time to me, and also ensured I had no difficulty attending appointments.

I found St Luke's Hospital and the Dublin Dental Hospital to be places of extraordinary sanctuary and the fact that St Luke's dealt exclusively with cancer was a great comfort. There was never any need to ask other patients why they were there.

The removal of some borderline-healthy teeth felt a bit strange; the extractions and the fluoride baths etc. kept me busy. They needed to be done and also passed the time and tempered my frustration while waiting for the manufacture of my mask for radiotherapy, which was probably the most frustrating wait of all. Other frustrations included the reticence of the VHI to sanction payment for a PET scan until after the event, so I had to fund it myself.

The best advice was probably the suggestion from a consultant general surgeon friend that I have a feeding PEG put in should swallowing become a major issue, which of course it did. Issues with swallowing led to my hospitalisation for six or seven weeks through Christmas, at St Luke's.

The pain endured, the treatment with a morphine pump, the weaning-off and come-down from morphine are now distant memories, as if they were things that happened to someone else. But those memories will remain with me for ever. At this time I was not capable of depression or anxiety. To an extent I felt I was losing my grip, but I never thought I was dying. I think I was acting like a well-behaved prisoner who was happy to get into a cocoon and undergo a rollercoaster ride of treatment for whatever reason, always believing that I would survive.

In the hospital I had no appetite for visitors except for family and my own inner circle, and I had no difficulty sleeping in their presence or suggesting that a successful hospital visit for the patient should last no longer than 20 minutes. Reintegration into home, my community and, gradually, work, while not difficult, felt eerie and had an inexplicable element of guilt for me.

Learning to taste again in April 2006 when the PEG was removed was difficult. Soft or supposedly fairly innocuous things like melon tasted very acidic and I could only positively identify my favourite food, potatoes, by texture and vision.

Products for dry mouth bought over the internet from the US were of no benefit. Over the years I have become more tolerant of hot food; garlic and the like induce serious dry mouth, as do stressful situations. My wife was always interested in food and there are no special recipes but she was able to cater for my need for inoffensive food.

My main residual problem is the almost total loss of hearing in my left ear from the radiotherapy, which has resulted in numerous minor operations and consequent difficulties with crowd noise, music and danger crossing roads as I now hear noise from the opposite direction.

I have no real dental problems which I attribute to the care advice and encouragement I continue to get in the Dublin Dental Hospital. Now the whole family uses interdental brushes, which has saved us a few bob!

I don't believe there are silver linings to cancer. But I do feel that I got a second chance. All the promises that I made that I would never work as hard again have been broken because of a mixture of on the one hand feeling lucky that I can work at all, and on the other the recession leaving me in a position where I must work extraordinarily hard to survive, which in itself is stressful.

I don't think I am a complete hypochondriac as a result of cancer but I think I was off the air for about a year almost completely, and that my recovery has been in a positive direction since. Largely I am now in good health, with no fear of dying, and I – selfishly – hope not to outlive those I care for.

———•———

Bernie Dwyer

THIS IS THE STORY I wasn't going to write. I've told the story hundreds of times but I held back from writing it down. Lots of people suggested that I keep a diary of my treatment and recovery and I went as far as buying a very posh diary with a colourful cover, to keep notes. After three days I was bored with it. But when this project presented itself, I thought the time was right to put my experience down on paper.

I was working as a radio journalist in Havana, Cuba, when I became aware of a swelling on the left side of my neck. I had a biopsy done, which came back negative. I was also referred for a lung X-ray and mammogram both of which proved clear. Soon afterwards the lump disappeared and I forgot about it.

I had done everything I could, hadn't I?

Not long after that I became very conscious of a growth at the back of my throat. For a while, it was a minor irritant but soon it became very uncomfortable to swallow. I went back to the hospital and had several biopsies done.

In 2006 I was diagnosed with cancer of the tonsil after 18 months of going to public and private hospitals and specialists in a developing country. Apparently the sophisticated equipment to read the biopsies just wasn't available.

So, back in Dublin, I went to an ENT specialist who looked at the medical files I had and said that maybe I should have a scan, which I did. Then I got a phone call from him to tell me I had an appointment with an oncologist in St Luke's Hospital. The word cancer wasn't mentioned but the clues were there. I went to St Luke's to be told I had a stage 4 squamous tumour and that I had a 70 per cent chance of survival. I remember saying to myself that I am going to be in the 70 per cent.

So my treatment started very soon after that. I had radiation and chemotherapy over several months. I started the radiation in a very positive frame of mind, as for a while there were no uncomfortable effects. But then I was admitted as a patient to St Luke's Hospital as my oncology doctor upped the treatment to twice a day. It was then that the effects began to kick in. The biggest discomfort was that I was fed through a tube in my nose, as my throat couldn't cope with swallowing anything. The skin on my neck was burning and it was so bad that I was self-administering morphine to try to keep the pain away.

Just as the treatment was finishing up I found a lump in my left breast. I was sent from St Luke's to Beaumont Hospital for a scan, and there it was – a lump that had to be biopsied. It was malignant and I went to see the breast cancer specialist in Beaumont. He explained that I would have to have a mastectomy.

Back in St Luke's, I had to finish my radiation treatment.

On 13 December I had my mastectomy and I woke up the next day, my birthday, in a ward in Beaumont. I was discharged on 15 December as there was a virus alert in Beaumont.

I live on my own, so I was lucky to have a friend who moved in to nurse me, as I still had the draining cups attached to the surgical site.

It's amazing how the mind deals with pain. Whereas I know I suffered severe pain during all these procedures – chemotherapy, radiation and surgery – I can't quite reach it in my mind now.

The final effects of radiation on my throat made swallowing difficult. This meant that I had to eat food that was soft and easily swallowed. That was a nuisance as I was constantly choking on pieces of chicken, the only meat I allowed myself. I finally copped on to the fact that I couldn't swallow chicken. I became a vegetarian, as that was the simplest option.

When it was all over I remember thinking that I hadn't realised how much I was loved by my family and friends. They were suffering as well but kept it very much between themselves so as not to upset me. Those of us with families are certainly blessed because of all the love and support they bring us at a time like this.

The main thing I learned from this experience is not to ignore any signs that might point to tumours or unusual growths. If the first doctor doesn't refer you to a specialist go and get a second opinion. I wasted too much time taking the easy way out and going on my merry way as soon as I was told it wasn't anything to worry about.

Once I was in the medical system the care and medical attention I received from the doctors and nurses in St Luke's and Beaumont Hospital was nothing less than stupendous. Also I couldn't have done without the dentists and students in the Dublin Dental Hospital. They made my life much easier at a time when I was still getting to grips with the fact I had cancer. It's so easy to slip into denial about the reality that one is suffering from a serious disease.

I had six years' remission but unfortunately the cancer returned in 2011 with tumours on my tongue. This time I had to have very serious surgery to remove two thirds of my tongue. So life wasn't too easy after that as I also have a tracheostomy, which means that I have to feed myself through a tube in my stomach. There's no doubt that my life is not so simple now but if I organise myself well I can go to the cinema and theatre or family events.

A year later tumours in my mouth returned and I am receiving chemotherapy in Beaumont Hospital at the moment. Let's hope that all turns out well. I am delighted to have the opportunity to write my story about my experience of cancer of the mouth and throat, which I hope is useful to those reading it.

This project has certainly helped me to write it down, posh diary or not.

Ann McCaffrey

IN JUNE 2002 I WAS a perfectly health 52-year-old woman, married with four daughters. My eldest daughter had just sat her college exams and my youngest had just completed her Leaving Cert. The middle two girls were attending college in Galway. I worked as a part-time staff nurse in St John's Community Hospital, Sligo. I had noticed my left tonsil was enlarged for some time, but it was not causing any problems.

One day I felt a lump under my left jaw and went immediately to my GP. I also told him about my tonsil. When he examined me he said I probably had chronic tonsillitis and gave me a prescription for a ten-day course of penicillin. The day I completed the antibiotics I returned to my doctor who referred me to one of the ENT consultants in Sligo General Hospital. Two days later I saw him in his private rooms. After a detailed history and examination he made arrangements for me to have a biopsy of the lump and my tonsil removed the following morning.

On discharge three days later, arrangements were made to return to the clinic at Sligo General for the biopsy results. Even though I suspected what the diagnosis would be, I was shocked when I was told it was malignant, and a wave of panic came over me. I thought my life was over. The nurse and consultant tried to reassure me, but I still went home in a daze. It was the only thing I thought about for the rest of the day, and I wondered how I got it. Later on that evening I told my family the results. Over the next week or so I told friends; they were shocked but they were a great support.

About two weeks later I saw the visiting oncology team in Sligo Hospital. After being examined I was told how my treatment would proceed. I was told to try to put on weight and take supplementary nutritious drinks between meals and before bedtime. An appointment was made for me in the Dublin Dental Hospital, which I attended in August. My treatment started in St Luke's Hospital, Dublin in mid-September, about seven weeks after meeting the team. All aspects of the treatment were explained to me. I was also informed of the side effects and I was anxious that I would not be able to cope with them.

About a week or so into the treatment my throat and mouth got very painful and my swallowing got very difficult. I was given pain relief about half an hour before meals, with some effect. My appetite diminished and I also began vomiting. I started losing weight and I became dehydrated. I was commenced on intravenous fluids and supplementary feeds via PEG tube, which was inserted straight into my stomach through my tummy.

The level of pain intensified and the pain relief I was given was no longer effective. I was commenced on a syringe driver. This is a method of giving a continuous flow of medication and it greatly reduced the pain. Nine weeks after admission my treatment was completed, and I was discharged on PEG feeds and oral pain relief.

I was told to visit my ENT consultant as soon as possible to make arrangements for surgery on the left side of my neck. I was referred to an ENT consultant in Dublin who performed a left-sided neck dissection three weeks after my discharge from St Luke's. The surgery involved the removal of the muscle, glands and nerves in my neck, resulting in my left shoulder drooping and an inability to raise my left arm. The nerve that enables swallowing was also removed. This resulted in me being unable to swallow food normally. I could only take a liquidised diet, with plenty of fluids to help me swallow. My salivary gland was also removed, leading to dry mouth. I had to take very frequent sips of water to keep my mouth moist. A week after surgery, I was discharged.

Mealtimes at home were a big problem, trying to make nourishing sloppy food. Initially my diet was mostly milk-based. A small amount of Weetabix with hot milk, semolina, mashed banana, yoghurt, cream cheese mixed in soft mashed potatoes, scrambled eggs and tinned salmon mashed with mayonnaise. Eating was very slow and laborious; I took up to an hour to eat very little. Overnight I had a litre of liquid food via PEG.

Very slowly I added vegetables that I liquidised with stew, soup or gravy with a handheld blender. All during this time I had regular home visits from the community dietitian. She weighed me on each visit, encouraged me to eat, and made suggestions on how to make my food appetising and nutritious. Gradually my food intake increased and about six months after surgery I started to gain weight.

A year later the PEG tube was removed and I was discharged from the dietitian's care. During this time I was also attending the speech and language therapist in St James's Hospital, Dublin for swallowing exercises.

I am now back to my normal weight but continue to have swallowing problems and need a sloppy diet.

I completed my first mini marathon in June 2004, walking of course. I did a total of five over the following years.

I retired from my permanent nursing post at the end of 2004. My four daughters are now married and I have five beautiful grandchildren. Sadly none of them live in Sligo.

Today, ten years later, I am a perfectly healthy woman enjoying a full and active life.

My mouth continues to be dry, but has improved over the years; I always carry a bottle of tap water. When eating out I usually order fish and request extra sauce to mash my potatoes and vegetables.

Due to being unable to lift my arm high, I have to wear loose tops that can stretch, I put my left arm in first, manoeuvre my head into it, then put my right arm through. I wear dresses with a full-length zip so I can step in, pull the dress over my hips, then put my arms through. I have to get help with the zip.

Life is good.

Suggestions

Initially my food had to be liquidised to a very smooth purée. I did this with a handheld blender. Root vegetables are very easily puréed with a little gravy, sauce or milk. I did them separately so they looked more appetising. Meat was impossible to swallow so I used fish, fresh and tinned salmon mashed with mayonnaise. My fruit intake was tinned peaches, mashed. I also stewed apples, rhubarb, pears and plums and mixed them with custard.

———•———

Michael Keenan

CHELTENHAM FESTIVAL, 2006: WAR OF Attrition wins the Gold Cup by two and a half lengths. The crowd goes wild. I cast my mind back to a year earlier when I was watching the very same race and Kicking King romped home. Back then I was feeling unwell with a sore throat, cough and hoarseness. Even with my winnings in my pocket and plenty of Guinness flowing, the discomfort never diminished that day or indeed for a further two weeks.

Around Christmas 2005 I made an appointment to see my GP. My sore throat had returned and it felt like an army of midges dancing at the back of my throat. I had an earache on top of this. Over the next four months I was back and forth to the doctor, who prescribed four different antibiotics.

Move forward again to Holy Thursday 2006. I woke one morning to find three lumps on my neck. I was very concerned. I got an appointment to see an ENT Consultant and after his examination he was able to confirm I had tonsil cancer. I felt profoundly sad and upset to hear the news but I was also relieved as I now had an explanation for what was wrong with me. He advised me that I was in for a tough time – nine to 12 months give or take of it – and how right he was.

Watching War of Attrition run that race, little did I know how apt this name would be to my recovery. By definition, a war of attrition is a struggle in which you harm your opponent in a lot of small ways, so that they become gradually weaker. This was what had been happening for the past year and now that I had identified my enemy, there was no way I was going to give up without a damn good fight. I was glad that I had stopped smoking two years before as it meant I didn't have to deal with the stress and withdrawal symptoms of quitting on top of everything else.

Surgery

I was admitted very quickly to the ENT ward of the Mater Public Hospital. Oddly enough for the first time I felt relaxed and secure. The care I received was second to none. They made me feel important, spoiled even, by all their attention. I was comfortable and had wonderful support from the staff there. Above all else, I knew I wasn't in this battle alone. I had a team of soldiers and generals planning a strategy for my recovery. I knew I was in the best of hands.

I was to spend three weeks in hospital where blood tests, X-rays and other tests were a daily part of my stay. It was explained to me that the cancer originated in my tonsil and that it was not possible to surgically remove it. The cancer had spread from my tonsil to the lymph nodes in my neck but thankfully had not spread beyond there.

I had surgery to place a feeding tube in my stomach, and to remove those lymph nodes from my neck. The surgery was quite extensive and I was advised to build myself up over the next month or so, prior to embarking on the next phase of my treatment. I recuperated at my sister's house and felt strong heading into the next phase. The tonsil cancer itself was to be treated with an intensive course of daily radiotherapy and weekly chemotherapy over the next few months.

Radiotherapy

The radiotherapy was to be directed at a small area. In order to reduce the damage to healthy parts of my neck, a special mask was made, which I wore during the radiotherapy sessions. It was difficult to sit so still for between ten and 30 minutes per radiotherapy session, but tolerable overall. We drove to the Mater Hospital every day Monday to Friday for the radiotherapy treatment.

As the radiotherapy continued I began to feel more and more tired. The radiotherapy began to cause some local complications and it caused the skin to peel around the site of the wound on my neck. Swallowing, which was already a problem, became more difficult as the radiotherapy dried up saliva production in my mouth. Nausea came later and only occurred for the last ten of those radiotherapy treatments.

I was losing weight and I felt pretty miserable towards the end of the radiotherapy, to be honest. The cancer itself, the surgery and now the radiotherapy were taking a toll on me. I was very much a wounded soldier, but I knew I still had a battle to fight. It was very hard at times.

I reflect on this particular phase of my treatment a lot as I found this the toughest. My wife has progressive MS and with the best will in the world from her and my children it was not possible for me to be cared for at home at this point. I stayed with my sister and her husband and they provided invaluable care and support to me, for which I will always be so grateful. I wonder at times, though, if it would have been more appropriate to have been an inpatient for that part of the treatment as intensive nursing care is invaluable and very reassuring at this very vulnerable part of the journey.

Chemotherapy

I had chemotherapy once a week throughout the course of the 38 sessions of radiotherapy. I lost three stone of my body weight in that time. I was unable to eat, drinking was very difficult, and speaking was painful. My mouth was very, very dry. The feeding tube that was placed in my stomach prior to treatment was invaluable and provided me with much needed nutritional support. The PEG feeding was not all plain sailing, though. It took some getting used to, and some help from family members daily to set it up for me.

I knew at this point I was at the mountain peak, my treatment was over and I was in the recovery phase of my illness. There was light in sight.

Recovery

Complications were to follow. Some were to be expected but others not so and unfortunately I developed osteoradionecrosis (see Medical Terms) of my jawbone as a result of the radiotherapy. I had already been attending the Dental Hospital for dental care pre- and post-treatment, but I was to become part of the furniture there over the next number of months and years as they tended to the many dental and oral problems that arose.

My teeth were affected by the radiotherapy, but they were not great to start with. We decided to go down the route of upper teeth implants. The Dublin Dental Hospital was of the opinion that my health and mouth were strong enough to withstand the planned treatment and surgery I would have to face. After two years of dedicated treatment by the dental staff I am happily smiling again and my confidence has returned. They deserve nothing but praise and credit for the part they play in the recovery and after-care of all ENT patients.

With the support of my team, family and friends, the whole experience of cancer and my road to recovery has been a positive one, if I can say that. At no time did I feel I was alone in this. The support I received was exceptional –

crucial on my journey and invaluable in my recovery. I will be forever indebted to all the wonderful people who have cared for me along the way. A patient does not journey through a cancer diagnosis and treatment on his own; his family journey with him. It takes a huge toll on both patient and all those who care and love them. It is an emotionally exhausting journey, but one that teaches you what really matters. It did this for me and I am ever so grateful to have been given a second chance. I know how lucky I am.

A positive attitude is crucial to recovery. You have to focus, not on what has happened and what you can no longer do, but rather on all the opportunities open to you. I had a few sessions of reiki through the ARC Cancer Support Centre, which I found very beneficial. They have been a great support and the ENT nurse has been exemplary.

In my period of recovery I have learned how to use a computer and have been taking piano lessons for the past four years. I am back playing golf after two years away, and I'm playing better than ever! I am now a grandfather to six wonderful grandchildren and to spend time with them and see them grow is the best thing I could have wished for. I have regained the weight I lost and am enjoying life. As I sign off on my story I am two days post-surgery. I was admitted briefly for an oesophageal dilation procedure (see Medical Terms) and look forward to seeing a big improvement in my eating and swallowing.

Good luck to you all in your recovery.

———•———

CANCER OF THE PALATE (HARD AND SOFT)

Stefan Sipka and Natalia Sipkova

I HAD BEEN UNEMPLOYED FOR QUITE some time. I wasn't sure what was going on with me until my daughter Natalia translated everything for me. I do remember my wife was over one night with my daughter and she rang up for an appointment for me to see a dentist. I had a bad smell in my mouth and I had problems with swallowing. When the dentist checked me out in Ongar I was referred to the Dublin Dental Hospital for examination and that's how it all started. I was told in the Dublin Dental Hospital there was something growing in my mouth and it looked like a mushroom. They took a sample of it and I was told to wait for the results.

After a few days I got a letter from the Dublin Dental Hospital. I couldn't understand anything. I waited until my daughter came in from work and I asked her to read it and explain it to me. I could see from her face that she wasn't sure what it was about. She told me she would take the letter to her boyfriend's mum and read it to her. Next day when my daughter came she said, 'Dad,' and at this point I knew something wasn't right, 'you have cancer in your mouth. You are being referred to St James's Hospital to see some special doctors.'

I am a very strong person, so I said, 'I know I will be fine,' but inside I wanted to cry. In the next few days everything was as usual. We got a letter to go and see a consultant in St James's Hospital. It all went so quick, that I didn't have time to think about it. My cancer was so big that they wanted to do the surgery very fast.

My surgery took 11 hours. When I woke up I remember I couldn't move and I was sweating everywhere. My head was like a balloon. They cut my neck open and I had tubes inside it, for breathing. They also cut my face because my cancer had spread to my cheek and they had to remove it. They also took skin from my leg to cover my palate. I was in the hospital for three weeks. I had my neck stapled after surgery, as stitches would not hold it together.

I was recovering pretty well. I couldn't talk properly for some time and it's still the same. I was told before surgery about all the side effects. All the doctors and nurses were so good. I cannot say a single bad word about them.

After three months of recovering I had a scan to see how I was doing. I was told there was something left, so I needed to have radiotherapy for six weeks and some chemotherapy as well. I took everything very easy.

Before my treatment started I had to have my teeth checked out and all the weak teeth taken out, because radiotherapy will damage your teeth.

My treatment started on 5 September and lasted for six weeks in St Luke's Hospital. I had to have a mask made to protect my face. The first two weeks were fine. I wasn't sore or anything, just my face was getting red. In the middle of the third week I started feeling tired and in pain. I was seen by nurses almost every day and by a doctor every Wednesday. I had a tough time.

Everything was organised in the hospital. I had transport from the hospital every day. Everybody was trying to help me. There was a language barrier, so they all tried very hard. Many times they had to ring my daughter Natalia, because I couldn't understand at all. There was never any issue with anything at all.

After my treatment I was so tired. I used to sleep for days. My neck and face were numb. My mouth was like the Sahara. So dry. It's still the same. I can't eat or drink properly. I can't go out for a meal because I can't swallow solid food. I can eat soups or yoghurt smoothies. I am very thirsty all the time. I drink so much – fizzy drinks, juices and water too.

A long time after my radiotherapy finished, my teeth went bad and became painful. I went to my dentist and had some of my teeth taken out. After this I got an infection in my jawbone called osteoradionecrosis (ORN). My daughter took me back to the Dental Hospital and I am still having treatment there for the exposed bone and the pain.

My whole life changed. I will never be able to do things like before. My wife is trying so hard to put up with me and I know sometimes I am like a different person. It's hard to live like this but I hope I will live as long as I can.

It's two years now since I was diagnosed with mouth cancer. I feel better after my treatment. I can feel my neck and mouth. I still struggle with dry mouth and eating. Whatever I eat I feel like I have sand in my mouth. My daughter is always beside me. I would never talk about my cancer with anybody. I am trying to live my life happily. I am still smoking. I know it's killing me but I can't stop and it's giving me some kick for my bad days.

———•———

RK

I THINK ONE OF THE biggest challenges for me early on was just to get over the initial shock and accept that I had cancer. I didn't feel sick. As far as I was concerned I was young and healthy. It couldn't be cancer.

In the run up to diagnosis I hadn't had too many issues with my mouth. I had a swelling on the roof of my mouth after having work done on my front teeth, but this settled down and wasn't painful. I wasn't concerned. When I eventually went to get it checked out it was more to make sure everything was okay than out of a fear that something was wrong.

My dentist referred me to a periodontal specialist in the Dublin Dental Hospital and I was seen quickly by her. It was only when a biopsy was taken that I started to get a little concerned, but I never really feared cancer; I was 22 and in college, it couldn't be cancer. So when the diagnosis was given I couldn't really get my head around it. It never really sank in until I was in hospital.

Everything moved quickly after diagnosis; before I knew it I was in hospital preparing for my first operation. My main issue was the swelling after the surgery. It took a few days for it to start to settle down, and even after that I couldn't eat or drink anything other than water for two weeks, which can be frustrating on the ward when everyone around you is getting three meals a day.

But all the swelling and pain post-surgery eventually settled and after a few weeks I was fitted with my first obturator/denture (see Medical Terms). It was uncomfortable at first and difficult to get used to, but really not that bad. You learn to adapt and eat with it, and once you get used to the feel of it, it's fine.

I was lucky in that I didn't have to undergo any radiotherapy etc. post-op, and this undoubtedly helped in my recovery. But I think the most important thing that helped me was staying positive. Instead of focusing on how I was too young to have cancer, I focused on how much time I still had ahead of me. Having cancer had a huge impact on my short-term plans but I wouldn't let it affect me in the long-term. It's one of toughest experiences of your life, but it passes. And when it's over you look back and realise that you're stronger for it.

Suggestions

- ➤ Make short term goals
- ➤ After surgery, make goals for yourself to achieve at the different stages of your recovery. It makes it easier to mark progress and gives you something to focus on. For example, I focused on walking further distances each day to build up my strength again
- ➤ Be open
- ➤ Build up a network of people close to you who you can talk openly with about how you're getting on. It's much easier to talk to someone about problems you might be having when they've been with you every step of the way

Sandra Keating

I WAS 57 WHEN I was diagnosed with carcinoma of the palate, five years ago. My family were reared (three sadly emigrated) and I had a full-time job. I already had angina and a stent, high cholesterol and blood pressure problems, so I was used to dealing with medics, hospital visits etc.

I'd had about six months of bleeding gums, recurrent coldsores and mouth ulcers before noticing white patches and something on my gum before going to my dentist. I worked in a library, and had done some research. I'd guessed I was in trouble though I knew nothing about mouth cancer – this was before the recent mouth cancer awareness campaign. Back then I knew nobody who'd had it, but this month alone I have heard of two new diagnoses locally. I had given up smoking ten years earlier, had an occasional glass of wine, and never drank spirits. My dentist confirmed that I had leukoplakia (see Medical Terms) and referred me to a periodontal surgeon but I was on a six-month waiting list to see him. He then referred me to the Dublin Dental Hospital and again I was put on a six-month waiting list. I should have pursued faster appointments through my dentist or GP, as I found when I was finally admitted to St James's that my 'ward buddies' had all had their appointments fast-tracked.

During my initial treatment in the Dublin Dental Hospital, before I was diagnosed, the leukoplakia was treated with creams but to no avail. Once I started experiencing pain, my gum lesion was biopsied. I was told I would be hospitalised quickly and tests and scans would be done to see if 'it' had spread. Rather naively, I had never thought of this. I was in for over a week before the operation, having a test a day – bloods, MRI, CAT, PET. This was five years ago; I doubt I'd be 'blocking' a hospital bed for so long these days!

I saw the speech therapist and dietitian before the operation, but I really had no idea how difficult speech and eating were going to be initially, though they emphasised that, because it was the palate, I 'might wake up with nothing between my tongue and my nose'.

I suppose I was in denial. I just could not imagine this, and in the event it was nothing like as bad as that, but medics do tend to give worst-case scenarios and it's probably just as well. In the event, the operation was long, as I had a triple haemorrhage. Then I was trying to sleep sitting up, while connected to transfusions, drips etc, with blood oozing from my nose for a week, a mouth full of obdurator, pain, a diet of sickly, sweet drinks and Yops, drooling, drooling, drooling and the usual hazards of hospital existence: constipation, insomnia, boredom, too-loud TV's and patients who refused to wear headphones. It was lovely, though stressful, to see family and friends, as I looked hideous and they found it hard to understand me.

Desperate to get out of hospital, I gibbered with fright when told I could go home. I had little support; how would I cope? So the weeks passed slowly. I was lonely and exhausted. The infections came thick and fast, but I was not allowed more antibiotics (and proper order!). Difene for the pain gave me diarrhoea. I weaned myself off painkillers so I could drive again (I had a muzzy head from all the drugs). I tried to do my mouth exercises, but it was so hard to open my mouth.

The weakness and fatigue became depressing. The consultant would chuckle to the team in Outpatients: 'Here she comes with her list of questions, and the first one will be "Why am I so tired?"' But it is vital to ask questions and in fairness I usually got patient answers. But the tiredness never went away. And the gagging and choking are still a problem – beware string beans, lettuce, rocket, bread crumbs! But the first unshredded apple was a triumph! The road to recovery seemed very slow, though I suppose it's the same for all cancers. But I think mouth, head and neck cancer is so visible and obvious that it seems harder.

I went back to work after five months – probably too soon, but I would have gone off pay. I still only work half-time as I get so tired, so I come home, have a rest, recharge and am ready to go again. I have to pace myself. I was very lucky I did not need chemotherapy or radiation. I am not one of those lying loo-lahs who say they are glad they got cancer because it changed their lives, but I do seize the day. I get out in the fresh air every day and listen to nature, and though I'm not religious, I am thankful to have come through and that I am so well. I think of the Indian proverb: I turn my face to the sun and let the shadows fall behind. From it all, I will never forget the astonishing tsunami of love that washed over me from family and friends, which bore me up and through my cancer. Every call, letter, poem, prayer, text, card, present – all were treasured. Support means so much. Finally, the health service lurches from crisis to crisis – diamonds and rust; the staff are the diamonds.

Suggestions

> Warm saltwater mouthwashes for mouth ulcers. Raw clove of garlic rubbed on first sign of coldsores on lips, and use a tea-tree stick

> A spoon of good Manuka honey per day held in the mouth till it dissolves. Good active UMF New Zealand honey is very expensive but very good[3]

---

3. Manuka honey may have value, however it should not be allowed to rest in the mouth for too long or be taken too frequently or it will cause dental decay.

- ➤ Green tea for antioxidants. Also dark berries, especially blueberries, in smoothies
- ➤ Laughter is the best medicine. Dance; close the curtains, put on Joe Dolan and dance

Books I found helpful

- ➤ Lia Mills's book *In Your Face* made me laugh and cry. It was my story too (in lots of ways)
- ➤ *Cancer is a Word Not a Sentence* by Dr Robert Buckman
- ➤ *Take off Your Party Dress* by Dina Rabinovitch. The story of a woman too busy to have breast cancer. She writes about how we must endure the misery and start our lives over

————◆————

CANCER OF THE OROPHARYNX

Reginald MacMahon

I HAD TAKEN EARLY RETIREMENT at the age of 56 and I was enjoying a very active retirement. One could say I was having a life that presented no cares whatsoever. I was six years into retirement when over a long period of time – say six months – I began experiencing recurring sore throats.

Initially the various antibiotics that were prescribed did appear to be of some benefit, but as time passed it became apparent that they were having no effect whatsoever. Eventually, my pharmacist felt that the recurring throat problem should be investigated further and it was he who suggested that I get a second opinion, as he was anxious that antibiotics should no longer be prescribed until I received another medical assessment.

I immediately took the pharmacist's advice because I was now experiencing a continuous soreness, especially when eating. I was conscious of the fact that I could no longer swallow my food in comfort. An ENT consultant performed an endoscopy while I was under anaesthetic and discovered that I had a tumour adjacent to the vocal cords.

I was informed that the tumour was at an advanced stage. The consultant in question referred me with great urgency to another consultant who had a more specialised knowledge of this particular type of tumour.

Because of the advanced stage of my tumour, time was of the utmost importance and a treatment programme was hurriedly scheduled. It consisted of an intravenous infusion of chemotherapy once a week for seven weeks, along with a simultaneous radiation programme of 37 sessions, each one lasting nine minutes. Prior to undergoing this treatment it was imperative that any foreseeable dental problems were attended to immediately, as radiation treatment to the mouth and throat areas curtails all forms of dentistry for a considerable period of time.

Having never before heard of anyone being treated for my type of cancer, I saw myself as being somewhat unique, and consequently I felt that because I did not have one of the more common cancers, my possibility of benefitting from any treatment programme was somewhat slim.

However, I had to accept the fact that I had a rare cancer. Much as I tried, I failed to locate a survivor, and this was mentally most problematic, for I simply had no one with whom I could converse in a non-medical way. At this juncture I was struck with the fear that my condition might be terminal.

In the early days of the treatment programme it was not a difficult task for me to get to the treatment centre because I lived within an hour's drive, but after several treatment sessions I was becoming lethargic, and this was coupled with the fact that radiation under the jawline area resulted in skin problems, tenderness and a severe soreness. This, along with the swallowing difficulties, necessitated me being hospitalised.

I was then fitted with a PEG tube to receive nourishment and medication that would normally be orally administered.

Psychologically, in hindsight, I believe being hospitalised was good for me because I got the benefit of specialised nursing care from professionals who understood what I was experiencing: ongoing swallowing difficulties and the weakening of my speech to but a whisper. Additionally, a stiffness in the neck and shoulder area developed but this was to be expected because the tissues around my neck were reacting to the radiation treatment. This area now required specialised dressings each day, a painful procedure, which of course was considerably eased by pain-controlling medicines.

Throughout the treatment programme there was an ever-present feeling of anxiety, heightened by the fact that the tumour in question had me hospitalised because I could no longer swallow solid or liquid foods, was unable to speak except in whispered tones and had a general feeling of weakness.

At that stage of treatment I often wondered if I would ever return to the normality of everyday life as I had known it. I was constantly reminded of the seriousness of my condition by the difficulties I had with speech, the severe jaw stiffness that limited mouth opening, and the progressive reduction in the functioning of my saliva glands. It was, therefore, only to be expected that depression became a problem, for I was conscious of the fact that, being part of a family, I was the centre of a situation which daily I had to accept as being beyond my control.

The only consoling factor was that, although I had taken early retirement, this problem, whatever the outcome, would not result in bringing about financial concerns, a matter of particular importance in the case of any serious or progressive illness.

Another aspect of my treatment programme was the fact that radiation in the throat area brings about a potentially permanent side effect known as dry mouth because of the damage it causes to the salivary glands and subsequent reduction in the amount of saliva produced. However, there are a multitude of mouth sprays and mouth washes on the market, and whilst in my case the situation is still ongoing it is to a lesser degree when compared with what I contended with over the first two years post-treatment. I now no longer have to use sprays because I have found that sucking hard-boiled sugar-free sweets and occasionally chewing special sugar-free gum keeps the remaining salivary glands sufficiently productive during waking hours. I have had to accept that the radiation programme has resulted in my lower salivary glands becoming defunct.

Just days before my discharge from hospital I was given the good news that the tumour appeared to be zapped. However, for almost three months following my discharge I had to rely on being connected to a PEG tube pump for several hours each day to receive one litre of liquid nourishment, together with four to six packs of other fortified food supplements, which I would syringe through the stomach tube.

During this period I gradually started to sip ice cream, then graduated to thin yoghurts and soups and then, in what would appear to be a mighty progression, to a variety of pâtés, but no toast! Initially food had no discernible taste – I simply experienced ingestion without flavour because of the effect of the radiation on my taste buds. It took perhaps six months before true tastes were once again apparent, but longer again for some foods. The PEG tube was removed about six months into the recovery programme, because it was then becoming possible for me to swallow, albeit in small gulps, my daily food requirements.

Psychologically the greatest boost was to know that I could taste, chew, swallow and drink foods in an almost normal manner, as before, and it was only then that I was relieved of the daily anxieties and broad spectrum of hindrances that this cancer imposed on me.

I am now in a position to look back over a few years and with great joy express my gratitude to all those who cared for me throughout my cancer journey, particularly the medics who encouraged me to accept what one must undergo in a treatment programme. Today I see myself as being fully well again, but of course like others I must accept any handicaps, such as my ongoing saliva problems through dry mouth, coupled with some eating and drinking limitations, but such issues are little to have to contend with, particularly when there is always another who has greater health problems to live with.

In my endeavours to help others overcome some of the problems I encountered during the period of my diagnosis and early treatment days I have become a peer support group member of the Irish Cancer Society where we have been trained to help those who face similar health obstacles. The helpline nurses of the ICS source survivors like me to speak with and/or meet those who need support (see Resources and Contacts).

———◆———

Valerie Bailey (Carer)

MY BROTHER WAS DIAGNOSED WITH throat cancer in June 2012. His problem began in April of that year when he started to have pain and difficulty chewing and swallowing on his right hand side. There was slight swelling, but it wasn't that visible externally. He went to his GP, who prescribed antibiotics but advised him to go straight to A&E if there was no improvement after three days. It took two visits to A&E, a month apart, before a CT scan showed a tumour above the right tonsil. A biopsy was taken the following week, and we had to wait two weeks for the results.

Then our worst nightmare came true: the tumour was malignant. It was decided the best course of action for a positive outcome would be 35 sessions of radiotherapy combined with three of chemotherapy. The success rate was better than 50 per cent.

My brother and all of our family were devastated by the diagnosis. Cancer is such a scary word and this was the first diagnosis in our immediate family, but we clung on to the fact that he had a good 50 per cent chance of recovery. At the time of diagnosis my brother was in a lot of pain, so painkillers were prescribed, which included morphine. It took a few weeks to manage, but with the help of the pain control team in St Vincent's Hospital, who were fantastic, the tumour pain eased off.

I always imagined that when cancer was diagnosed, treatment started straight away, but it's not as simple as that. Treatment requires careful planning and especially so with mouth, head and neck cancer. But everything fell into place very quickly. A couple of days after diagnosis we had an appointment with the radiation oncologist, who went through the possible side effects during and after treatment; we were told the worst-case scenarios that day, but thankfully they didn't happen.

The next appointment was a dental check-up in the Dublin Dental Hospital; this is essential before treatment. Our next appointment was with the oncologist who discussed the treatment and possible side effects of chemotherapy. I was surprised to discover that in my brother's case the side effects of radiation would be much tougher than those of chemotherapy. I always thought that chemotherapy was a much harsher treatment.

We had some good news that day – the PET scan my brother had a few days earlier showed the cancer hadn't spread to any other area. The next step in the planning was the making of a mask which had to be worn during radiation; this is necessary to keep you as still as possible.

My brother found the making of the mask really difficult but once treatment started he became accustomed to it. At this stage I decided that, because my brother was living alone, I would reduce my working hours. My employer was very supportive. I knew he was going to need lots of support to get through the treatment and beyond.

Treatment began approximately four weeks after diagnosis. After the first week my brother was quite unwell, mainly with dehydration, so he spent one week in hospital, then came home for a week, then went back in again and spent the final four weeks of treatment as an inpatient. About four weeks into treatment, because of weight loss due to difficulty chewing and swallowing, he had a PEG tube inserted. This was one thing my brother dreaded happening, but it was a lifesaver and wasn't as bad an ordeal as he had imagined.

In mid-September treatment finished and he was discharged from hospital. It would be 12 weeks before we would find out if the treatment was successful. In between we had appointments with the ENT team, the oncologist, the dentist and the dietitian. We also had visits from the district health nurse, so everyone was keeping a close eye on my brother's progress. My brother had a PET scan in early December and the results were good, showing no cancerous activity.

My brother had a few set-backs during the 12 weeks before results. He had a chest and mouth infection and a lot of jaw pain but he is recovering really well now. He had loss of hearing in his right ear due to fluid, but he recently had a procedure to rectify this and his hearing is perfect again. Dry mouth is a big issue and he carries a bottle of water constantly. He is eating again and his PEG tube is due to be removed shortly.

He has reduced mouth opening. This was caused by either the tumour or radiation. He is using wooden sticks several times a day to help stretch his mouth and is currently on a waiting list to see the speech and language therapist who will hopefully prescribe a TheraBite (see Medical Terms) which he feels will help him enormously.

He had some very dark days before and during treatment, but seven months on from diagnosis he is recovering very well, all thanks to his wonderful GP who advised him to go to A&E, and the fantastic care he received in St Vincent's Hospital, St Luke's Hospital and the Dublin Dental Hospital.

My brother was fortunate that he had a supportive family and wonderful friends who helped him through his illness. It's so important when a person is ill to have that level of support. I took on the role of carer when it came to medication, hospital appointments and helping him build up his strength again. He was self-employed and lost his business as a result of the illness, so there was a lot of form-filling and telephone calls to ensure some financial aid, which he was too ill to organise himself. My concern would be that patients without family support would fall through the net so I really hope the HSE have some kind of system in place to prevent this happening.

Publications I found helpful

I found the booklets from the Irish Cancer Society really helpful and found myself referring back to them many times before, during and after my brother's treatment.

———•———

CANCER OF THE NASOPHARYNX

Róisín Whelan

I WAS 19 WHEN I was diagnosed with cancer. It was the start of the summer and I remember all of my friends were packing up to go travelling and I was so jealous. I was staying at home, about to begin a very different journey that would change my life. People regularly ask what it was like to be told I have cancer. The truth is I don't remember much about that day. I was so sick for months leading up to my diagnosis, that the only thing I remember feeling was a sense of relief. Finally they had an answer and they were going to be able to put a stop to all of the pain I was in.

The symptoms had started a year before. I was exhausted all the time and slept for 14 hours a day. I went to get bloods taken to see if I was anaemic, but nothing showed up and my tiredness was put down to partying too much. The infection in my ear started and the pain was unbearable, but no amount of antibiotics could make it stop. Over time the pain got progressively worse and it began to spread down the left side of my jaw. I would wake up feeling paralysed and unable to open my mouth or to stand up, because the pain was too much to bear. A tablet containing ibuprofen and codeine was the only thing that got me through those hard days and I felt dazed a lot of the time.

One evening when I was working as a waitress, I realised that I couldn't hear. People were giving me their orders and I couldn't understand what they were saying. I had lost my hearing in my left ear and then shortly after that, I noticed a lump on the left side of my neck.

I was referred to a surgeon, who performed a biopsy, but the test results were inconclusive and I was subsequently referred to a haematologist in UCD, to see if I was allergic to something. He told me that I wasn't allergic to anything and that the likely cause of my symptoms was a tumour. I was referred back to the surgeon, who removed the swollen gland on my neck and he confirmed a few days later that it was cancerous (apparently the first biopsy didn't catch the cells). Immediately I was sent to an ENT consultant in St Vincent's Hospital and, following a hearing test, it was established that I had lost 85 per cent of my hearing in the left ear. He then stuck a camera up my nose and down the back of my throat and confirmed that I had a tumour in the back of my throat, right where my ear and nose connect. Nasopharyngeal carcinoma is a rare form of cancer that affects one in a million. Lucky me!

Everybody heard the news and of course they were shocked – no one expects a young girl to get cancer – but I was numb. I had got used to being in such pain that the diagnosis didn't register with me. I was in denial about the whole thing. It wasn't until I went to meet with my radiation oncologist that the reality set in. I was going to be treated with an aggressive course of radiotherapy and chemotherapy. I had heard lots of stories about chemo and radiotherapy, but never understood the processes, or how they affect the body.

I met with various people in the Dublin Dental Hospital and they went through the effects of treatment on the head and neck. One of the most common side effects of radiotherapy in that area is the damage to glands and muscles. They told me that the salivary glands would be affected and that there was a chance I would not be able to produce saliva again, which would result in my teeth becoming weak. Back in the hospital I had various scans and also had a mask fitted for treatment and the radiographer made a few ink marks on the mask, to make sure I was positioned correctly on the table. When you lie down the mask is placed on your face and fixed to the table so your head doesn't move during the radiotherapy treatment.

I received radiotherapy every day Monday to Friday at the same time for 12 weeks. A week into my radiotherapy treatment, blisters started to form on my tongue and I had a metallic taste in my mouth from the chemotherapy. Within two weeks my whole mouth was filled with blisters and by week four I was admitted into hospital. I was weak and tired and my throat was in agony, dry and raw from the lack of saliva.

Halfway through the treatment my hearing came back and my ear just popped, as if I had just got off a plane. The skin on my face and my neck was red and sore (just like sunburn) and my mouth and throat were so raw that I could no longer eat; I don't think I ate for the last ten weeks of treatment. I sipped water to combat the severe dry mouth and my voice was very hoarse and deep. I didn't sound like me. Coming to the end of my treatment, I got sicker and sicker. My hair began to fall out and the skin on my face and neck was so raw, that they had to use cling film to keep it protected when I had the mask on.

Within a few days of treatment ending, I began to feel slightly better. The skin on my neck was healing slowly and the blisters in my mouth were getting better. I even started to eat again after losing nearly 2.5 stone of weight. I started off with moist foods like Weetabix, then gradually moved on to mashed potatoes with gravy, and lots of ice cream; anything cold was very soothing on the throat.

My taste buds were all over the place and it took a year for them to return to what might be called normal. Roughly ten days after treatment ended, I had a scan, which confirmed they had got the tumour and I was in remission. The healing process was hard and it was difficult coming out of hospital after being there for so long. It took me a while to get back into real life and to reconnect with people after going through such a traumatic time. People told me I looked great because I had lost weight and I remember looking at them in disbelief, thinking to myself, *Do they not know what I have been through?*

Not only were the psychological effects hard to cope with, I also had to get used to the physical effects. My thyroid gland became inactive and I would have to take medication daily to combat the side effects. My saliva never came back and so I had to re-educate myself on the foods that were easy for me to eat. I could no longer eat spicy foods or even a bag of crisps, as I couldn't swallow without water. I had a bottle of water in my hand at all times and still do. Without the saliva protecting them, my teeth are now very weak. I am trying to manage it though. I don't drink fizzy drinks and I don't graze throughout the day. I keep all my eating to specific times, to counteract the acid. I chew sugar-free gum and I wash my teeth with a soft TePe toothbrush and special dry-mouth toothpaste. I use fluoride trays each night to help strengthen my teeth, and a mouth guard to stop the grinding. I drink a lot of water and I find taking little sips is most useful for keeping my mouth moist. Wherever possible, I drink tap water as it has fluoride in it, which helps keep my teeth strong. Most girls worry that their teeth aren't white enough, while I worry that one day I won't have any teeth!

This summer will be my tenth anniversary of the Big C. It's funny how time flies, yet I remember everything like it was last week. I can still smell the perfume the radiographer was wearing, hear the music playing on the radio going to the hospital, taste the metal in my mouth and feel that horrific pain in my face. I still have a great team looking after me in the Dublin Dental Hospital and I go to my oncologist every six months. For a week beforehand, I'm convinced that he'll tell me it's back and I have a cry. It's not until he puts a camera up through my nose and down my throat and says everything's fine that I finally breathe.

I have learned many things over the years about myself and cancer, but this is the one thing I'd like to share with people: the human body is strong and durable, but never underestimate the strength of the human spirit. And I think it was that that got me through those dark days.

———•———

Noel Reilly

IT WAS FRIGHTENING TO BE told the first time. I felt lost and that I had nowhere to go. I didn't know where to go or who to talk to. I had a hoarseness in my voice that my doctor noticed. Every second weekend, I'd be hoarse. That was it.

I went to the doctor with pain in the back of my legs, and he referred me to the ENT Department in the Mater Hospital because he noticed the hoarseness. The ENT people found something in my throat but they said it wasn't cancer. They got me to come back every so often for biopsies, and on the third biopsy, about two years after my first visit, they diagnosed a tumour on the back wall of my throat. The consultant said he couldn't operate because of where the tumour was. He referred me to St Luke's Hospital. I got 31 treatments with radiotherapy and two chemotherapy treatments.

I had heard of throat cancer, but I didn't know much about it.

Things that surprised me

➤ The loss of taste buds meant I wasn't able to taste food. It was like cardboard. My sense of smell went too

➤ How well they care for you in St Luke's. They just can't do enough for you. Even at four in the morning, they'd get you anything

➤ Transport was brilliant. I was picked up by a taxi at seven o'clock in the morning and brought to St Luke's every day when I was getting treatment

Challenges

➤ Trying to keep eating was a challenge, because of the lack of taste

➤ Lack of energy

➤ Depression came in for a while. At first, what comes into your head is that you'll fight it. After a month of fighting it, and not being able to eat, you get a little bit down and depressed. And then that got worse. I went very into myself

Silver linings

➤ The positive thing I got out of this experience was that having cancer doesn't mean you're going to die

Resources I found helpful

> ➤ The Acute Home Care Team in the Crannóg Unit in St Vincent's Hospital in Fairview

Food and diet

> ➤ The things I got a taste for were beans on toast and cream cakes. I was chasing the taste, as they actually tasted like cardboard. I put on weight chasing the taste

————◆————

Donna Gannon Bond (Carer)

MAM WAS THE LIFE AND soul of the family – hard working, great fun, always laughing. Her pet name is Mama Bear.

Mam started getting headaches and they became more and more frequent. She went back and forth to the doctor but always got the same diagnosis: migraine. Then overnight a gland on her neck swelled to the size of a small golf ball. More trips to the doctor followed, then antibiotics, and eventually a referral to St James's Hospital.

The biopsy done, 'Don't worry, Patricia, you should be fine,' was what she was told.

Three weeks went by. She had a check-up, and in passing she said, 'If I ring you, will you meet me?' Alarm bells went off in my head, but I suppose you block them out and I thought it was a routine appointment for something else.

The phone call came. 'I have your mother here; you need to come down,' the doctor said.

I don't remember that 15-minute trip to St James's Hospital; it's a blank.

The diagnosis was cancer. The lump was secondary, the doctor told me. This meant it was somewhere else too. Was it in the brain? Eyes? Mouth, or maybe the nose? Mam left the room. She didn't want to be there anymore; the word cancer was swimming in her mind.

I didn't tell Mam it was somewhere else until we had the full details. I felt she had enough to take in – one thing at a time. If the brain was mentioned she would have given up there and then.

My advice is: don't go on the internet. It puts fear and terror into your mind and confuses you even more.

Afterwards we got the full diagnosis. Thank God, it wasn't in the brain. It was behind the nose. And so our journey together began. Both our lives became so different.

Our first appointments were in the Dublin Dental Hospital, because Mam's radiation treatment would affect her mouth, teeth and gums. I can't tell you how nervous she was attending the Dental Hospital, I think everyone has fear going to the dentist. The staff and doctors in the Dublin Dental Hospital have been some of the most caring and helpful people I have met on this long journey. The way they spoke to Mam and took the fear away was great. Sadly Mam had to have her teeth removed. But won't she look lovely when she has her new teeth? Always a silver lining.

Radiation has been very severe on Mam. Dry mouth has to be the worst. She also has problems with swallowing and speech. Chemotherapy has affected her hearing.

Because of difficulties from treatment you have to be aware that you have to rebuild the person mentally and physically, and appointments are ongoing. Mam's immune system is very low, so infections are frequent, and what works for one person doesn't always work for another. Sometimes it's trial and error, but she keeps fighting on.

I suppose my biggest fear for Mam is her mind. Depression has set in and this is the hardest mountain to climb. Although Mam has won the battle against cancer she feels anxious all the time and is full of fear. Depression has really affected her, but the staff of St Luke's and St James's really work hard to help her fight this battle.

Life has changed because this disease affects the whole family in different ways and everyone has their own way of dealing with it. I think it's very important to tell the children in the family the truth and to keep them well informed. We didn't do this at the start and of course the children were picking up the wrong things, listening at different times to other people. It's really important to try to explain to the children as much as you can and let them ask as many questions as they need to ask, because they have the same fears as adults.

Mam is getting a little stronger day by day. It has been a difficult time in both our lives and for all the family, but you have to stay strong and positive, and that's why miracles do happen and we still have Mam – Mama Bear.

CANCER OF THE LARYNX

Philip McKeon

What symptoms did you have and how long did it take you to look for help?

A sore throat; about nine months.

Tell the story of your diagnosis and treatment

The cancer was discovered by accident. I was concerned about prostate cancer so I had a blood test. From the blood test they discovered my blood-sugar was very high. I was then sent to see the consultant endocrinologist in Loughlinstown Hospital. He asked me how long I'd had the sore throat and I told him about nine months, so he sent me to St Vincent's Hospital to see a specialist and he, in turn, did a biopsy.

The treatment was radiotherapy for seven weeks and I think one week of chemotherapy.

It was a shock at first, but I was reassured by the consultant that my condition was treatable. So I never worried after that.

What surprised you?

How reassuring the various doctors and consultants were.

Coordination of treatment

This was no problem. St Luke's Hospital organised everything.

Transport

Was no problem either. I live near Greystones, County Wicklow and it is only a short distance from St Luke's.

Fatigue

I did not feel any until after the treatment.

Pain

After about the third day my neck was getting quite painful, but the morphine soon cured that.

Eating

Big problem there. After a very short period of time into the treatment (maybe two days), I had no appetite at all and I was taking liquid food drinks. It took a while to get back to proper eating habits.

One thing was very helpful. A friend of mine is a chef and he worked for Ardmore Studios in Bray. Each day after treatment, I would drop in to my friend and he would insist I had to eat. I could not eat at the start, but what I did have was soup. So the first week I would have just a bowl of soup and then a little more soup, and by the end I would have three bowls of soup.

Speech

Obviously my speech was affected. My voice is high-pitched and I am used to that now, and the slagging I get from friends.

Swallowing

Swallowing was only a problem during the treatment and for a little time after.

Disfigurement

There is a scar under my chin and on my neck, so I just grew a goatee.

Mouth

I have no stiffness, but I do have reduced opening, which is no big deal.

Shoulder

I have a little neck pain if I turn a certain way, but again it's no big deal.

Fears

None at the moment.

Depression

I do think I went through a little depression during treatment, but I put that down to all the drugs I was taking because it stopped when the drugs stopped.

Family

My family were very supportive.

Financial

I worked for myself prior to treatment so I had some savings. I am not entitled to social welfare.

Dry mouth

That was a problem – drinking water all the time and going to the toilet quite a lot. Chewing gum is the answer for me, to generate saliva. In fact my dry mouth condition has improved.

Dental Problems

There are ongoing problems for me, I'm afraid. But with the help of the Dublin Dental Hospital, they are kept in check.

Silver lining

I was grossly overweight when I was first diagnosed. I lost weight very quickly and hopefully I can keep it off.

Resources

People, mostly in the Dublin Dental Hospital.

Diet

I do not have any recipes, but I do try to eat sensibly.

How are you now?

Mighty!

———•———

Martina Delaney

The Lump In My Throat

MY NAME IS MARTINA DELANEY and I am 55 years old, married with two grown-up children, a son and a daughter, and I also have one grandchild. Back in January of 2008, when I was grieving for my brother who had just passed away from liver cancer, I discovered a swelling on the right side of my neck. I had smoked for a short number of years in my late teens and early twenties, but once I gave them up managed to stay off them. I used to drink though. I suppose like a lot of young women these days I drank more than was good for me, but I was never a drunk.

The swelling was fairly painful and initially I thought it was just a gland, but when it didn't go away after a couple of weeks I decided to go to the doctor. At first he too thought it was glandular but he sent me for blood tests just in case. My blood tests came back clear but I was referred for a biopsy in order to investigate the swelling further. By this time I was feeling unwell in general with a lot of tiredness, and tightness in my throat was setting in. Within a few days, going back and forth to both James Connolly Memorial Hospital in Blanchardstown and the Mater Hospital, I was told that I had a cancerous tumour and would need surgery.

The day I was told is quite a blur but I do remember a lovely nurse gently placing her hand on my shoulder as the physician explained my prognosis. I felt the ground collapse under me when I heard the *C* word, but I remember thinking it would only be a matter of having the lump removed and I'd be fine. Yet deep down I knew it was serious and as I had lost both my brother and father to cancer I was also very worried.

The hardest part was telling my family. Even though they were young adults and I knew they were strong people, I still dreaded telling them and I must admit to putting it off for a few days until I came to terms with it myself. I remember when I did finally tell them we all huddled together like a bunch of penguins, all in tears and promising to beat it as a team! My daughter had previously had a very prophetic dream when she saw that the lump wouldn't be good news, and she had begged me non-stop to get it seen to after that.

I spent four weeks initially in the Mater having tests done in May of that year. They needed to find the primary source of the cancer through various scans and camera work; eventually they found that it originated at the base of my tongue of all places, deep inside my throat. So now the radiographers could pinpoint where to target the radiotherapy. I had a plastic mask made in order to facilitate the radiation treatment, which I was to receive down the line. It's a scary procedure and my mild claustrophobia initially almost brought on a heart attack every time I had it on. But as time went on I grew used to it, promising myself a little treat of some sort at the end of every session, like a magazine or a CD. You have to keep telling yourself that this is what's used as the ammunition in your war and just get on with it, I guess. Radiotherapy unfortunately kills some of the good cells as well as the bad cells, not unlike the good sometimes having to die along with the bad in any battle. This is when the saliva glands can get damaged but every care possible is taken to limit the long-term damage.

Treatment

In June after I had an operation called a neck dissection, during which I had the lump, gland and muscle removed, I was given my treatment plan, which would begin when I recovered at home and became strong enough again. I'd had a few setbacks with lymph fluids going haywire and having to be drained, but for the most part I got over the surgery fairly well. I remember waiting to be called in to start my treatment for those few weeks at home thinking, *Sure this is grand, I'll soon be right as rain!*

I had 35 doses of radiotherapy, five doses of chemotherapy and lots of medication for everything from pain to anxiety, including nausea.

At this point once again there was no place for me but hospital and I was admitted to St Luke's for a further four weeks in August. The radiotherapy affects the swallow and taste buds. I got endless mouth infections and became very depressed. I completely lost my appetite and swiftly went from a hefty 13 stone to just below nine in the space of a couple of weeks. I lived on PEG feeds and baby food. As time went on I progressed to soups, sauces, chocolate, yoghurts, jelly and ice cream but I could taste none of them.

During the time I was in the Mater before I had my surgery, I was sent to the Dublin Dental Hospital where I first met the wonderful staff there. I have always had the best treatment and care there. Before that, if I had been told there would be a connection between the lump on my neck and my teeth, or that I would be getting tube fed for the best part of a year, I wouldn't have believed it.

Gradually through the consultations with the Dublin Dental Hospital team, and also at workshops, I learned more about what lay in store for me after my treatment. I was given lots of advice, along with pamphlets and literature and little treats like a new toothbrush and toothpaste. Also many samples of mouthwashes and gels for dryness and infections. However, I think at the time I couldn't really follow or understand a lot of what was explained to me, not because it wasn't being very well explained, but because I was so unwell and still in shock at the realisation that I was in this position in the first place. I'm afraid a lot of it went over my head and my concentration was very poor.

I remember one day standing with my husband outside the Dental Hospital on Lincoln Place waiting for a taxi to take us back to the Mater and just bursting into tears because I was so overwhelmed.

During my treatment I used to picture a group of 'Power Rangers' busy at work trying to make me better. These were my doctors and my own inner healers. I had a favourite pair of red shoes which I wore on my chemo days and I used to click my heels three times like Dorothy and wish myself good luck, hoping for the best.

I was being prepared for the possibility of being left with little or no saliva, having my speech and swallow affected, having my taste buds killed, losing weight and being left with scarring, all from the evil cancer and a radiation treatment designed to save my life. It was enough to knock me for good but I still hoped against hope that I would be strong enough to get through.

I was advised (and it is a good idea) to have a 'second pair of ears' with me at all visits. It's equally hard on the close members of the family, but my husband carried me through all the way and when I went blank and was ready to give up he was always well tuned-in to get the information from the many doctors, nurses and dietitians involved in my treatment.

The last thing I wanted to do when I was so sick was have fillings done and trays fitted for the daily fluoride washes. I hoped the team could appreciate this. However, seeing pictures of teeth falling out and the damage that the lack of saliva and hygiene can do to the teeth shocked me, I must admit, into acceptance, and in time I formed good habits. Also, needless to say, at times at home the last thing I wanted to do was soak my teeth in the morning and again at night. But I knew that if I wanted to save my teeth it had to be done. Throughout my life on a scale of one to ten in looking after my teeth I would put myself at about six or seven.

I've got lots of fillings and two crowns, but I still in midlife have all my own teeth and so it's important to me to look after them even more now. The Gel-Kam fluoride wash that I use is very expensive so I presume it is doing some good, but I do think it's far too dear. I attend my own dentist in The Square Medical Centre, Tallaght for regular check-ups. I wash my teeth now three times a day and use flosses and interdental brushes along with mouthwashes and gels as I am prone to mouth ulcers. In fact I have to be careful that it doesn't become an obsession! At night I use either BioXtra or Oralieve enzyme gels for oral dryness and of course I can't go anywhere without a bottle of water.

When I got the all-clear in November 2008, again we huddled together (like the penguins) and cried, this time with relief. It had been quite the year – one I'd rather forget, really. Yet it was such an enormous reality and mortality check for me, it's one I won't forget for many reasons.

After I got the all-clear I was still rather weak and unwell and found it hard to really believe it was true. I must admit to running back to the hospital with lots of small issues that I convinced myself could become big. But tests and understanding put my mind at ease for the most part and the doctors and nurses always managed to relieve my stress.

It's really important to attend check-ups, as that's when any possible issues can be nipped in the bud. I am almost five years down the road now and thankfully still in the all-clear zone. I have blood tests done every couple of months and cancer check-ups are now annual, and my dental checks are every six months. On a couple of occasions I've been concerned about jaw pain and mouth soreness but after reassurance from the Dublin Dental Hospital team or my doctors at the Mater, my mind is at ease once again.

Needless to say life alters completely after cancer and the niggling worry that it will one day return is always present like a dark cloud. I don't drink alcohol at all now. Never got the taste back for it and don't want to either. But now I know that even if cancer does return, God forbid, with the great medical expertise available to me, I will be okay. I've had some scary moments with choking on account of my poor swallow, but I have learned to only eat what suits me and very slowly. Semolina and rice pudding are my favourites.

I've learned to live with my dodgy mouth, scarred neck, jaw pain and stiffness, tinnitus, blocked sinuses, dead shoulder, fatigue and bouts of depression. I'm glad to be alive and lucky to be here, thanks to the medical experts and the progress that has been made in treating illnesses like mine. It's not so long ago that I wouldn't have had a hope, I know. Both my father and brother were already deceased at my age. I hope from now on the only lump I get in my throat will be from tears of joy, and that was the case last year when my beautiful granddaughter Jasmine was born. I bless the day she came and I'm grateful that I was here to see her.

And I can tell you that if you are going through any type of cancer right now you are in good hands. Trust the people assigned to your care. Don't be afraid to express your feelings – they are all well equipped for dealing with any issue at all. Naturally in all life's journeys it's possible to run up against a difference of opinion from time to time but that's okay. Even the ships in the night run into each other at times.

I never asked *why me?* I'd been brought up to understand that anything is possible and everything is just around the corner in this life. But just as it is possible for me to get the Big C it is also possible for me to conquer it, and with the help of my 'Power Rangers' I did just that. I couldn't fault the health system here in Ireland. I think it's second to none and I feel I can never thank my medical and dental teams enough for my health and well-being today. I'd also like to thank all the other fantastic people I met during my illness and the domestic and care staff, and of course the patients. Even in my own sickness I marvelled at what people have to deal with on a day-to-day basis, both those suffering from cancers, some of which are extremely disfiguring to both body and soul, and those working in the field in general. Special thanks to my precious family and friends, too. And of course I thank God. I think between us all we won the war and you will too.

———•———

BUCCAL CANCER

Lia Mills

MY STORY BEGAN WITH A rogue wisdom tooth that made me bite my cheek, especially in my sleep. The cheek got sore and inflamed. I put up with this for a while, as you do, and then I went to a dentist, who removed the tooth. *Good riddance*, I thought.

Before long the sore area in my cheek was back and growing. I saw two dentists, over a period of about eight months, while the sore grew and spread. I thought it was a mouth ulcer gone mad. One of the dentists thought I was chewing my cheek again. The second thought I had erosive lichen planus, a stubborn condition that's notoriously hard to treat. He tried to treat it with steroid tablets, antibiotics and by replacing mercury fillings, but no joy.

In the end I went to my GP, who referred me to the Maxillofacial Unit at St James's Hospital in Dublin. By that time I couldn't stretch my mouth to a full yawn, I couldn't eat on that side, the pain in my cheek kept me awake at night and I had a hard lump under the angle of my jaw. They did a biopsy. A week later, I went back to get the results and was admitted.

My diagnosis was that I had a squamous cell carcinoma in my right cheek. Further tests would show that it was in my gums as well, and had spread to several lymph nodes in my neck. The treatment was radical surgery, followed by aggressive radiotherapy.

In surgery they removed part of my jaw and my cheekbone and the lining of my cheek. They replaced them with bone, skin and fat cells taken from my leg. A radical neck dissection removed the lymph nodes, nerve and muscle from the right side of my neck. Then they stitched and stapled me back together and sent me back to the ward via the Intensive Care Unit.

I had a tracheostomy. I breathed through one tube and was fed through another. I had to learn to walk again - not well enough, as it happened. My leg fractured later and I had to be readmitted to have it reset. I was in plaster and on crutches for months, which made the rest of my treatment hard to coordinate, but as a friend of mine said, that may have been a bonus because I literally had to sit still and rest, which I needed to do. Otherwise, I'd have been running around trying to pretend there was nothing wrong with me.

I had various complications: issues with medication, pain, infections, two readmissions, blood transfusions, but in the end I muddled through to the slow process of recovering and adapting to the new me.

It's tempting to gloss over all of this, but it's important not to, because it shows that even if you have a late diagnosis like mine, even if the treatment plan seems unimaginably extreme when you hear it first, people get through it every day, and there is life beyond it.

The challenges and issues you might have to face beyond treatment are the great unknown. No one can tell you what it'll be like, because no two people have the same experience. Some people face enormous difficulties, while others sail through it with no trouble at all. Most of us have some residual issues we learn to cope with. For me, it was definitely worth it, although there were times, going through it, when I wondered if it would be. But time was what I needed, and time was what I got. Seven years, now, and counting.

The most important things I'd say to someone who's facing into treatment are:

➤ Sometimes the treatment can seem to do more harm than the disease. Don't ever forget how aggressive and destructive the cancer would be if left unchecked

➤ Don't panic. It doesn't happen all at once. Take every single thing that comes along one step at a time, and break each step into manageable bits

➤ Statistics don't mean anything when it comes to individual cases. The statistics don't know you, or anything about your personal history, how healthy you are, what your diet is, what genetic factors are at play or what other stresses or motivators you're exposed to. Statistics don't know a single thing about luck

➤ I could say don't go on the internet, but you will. Be careful what sites you visit, and be aware that you don't have all the information you need to process the statistics you find. Some reasonable sites are listed in the reference section of this book

➤ Don't drive yourself mad wondering how you got this disease, or how different things might be if you'd caught it sooner. You can't change it now, and you'll need every scrap of energy for what's ahead

➤ Every small thing that you can do for yourself helps. Initially I could only manage to open my mouth wide enough for three tongue depressors, but I kept at it and slowly, one stick at a time, it improved. It's still not great, but every little helps, and it was a thing I could *do*. I hated being helpless

What surprised me

I felt as though I'd been sleepwalking through my life until the diagnosis shocked me awake to the blunt truth that life ends, whether we're ready or not. I was more than surprised by how hard it was to face that. It's not exactly news, but it's different when it's real.

I was taken aback to discover that my own response to everything that happened was fundamentally practical and optimistic. I'd fancied myself as a card-carrying pessimist and cynic, before.

And I was blown away by the loving, generous response of my family and friends.

Here's another thing: I used to have a pathological fear of two things – dentists and flying. We're talking full-on panic attacks here. The fear of dentists had to go, out of necessity and due to constant, extreme exposure to the cheerful efficiencies and great staff of the Dublin Dental Hospital. But when treatment was over and it was time to get on a plane again, I was astonished to discover that I'd lost my fear of flying.

Outcome

I am mostly well today. I have less energy than I used to and I'm less able to concentrate. I have issues with pain, deafness and tinnitus on that side, Frey's syndrome, restricted mouth opening and tongue mobility, and related problems with speech and eating, although I can usually manage (I like to think) so that other people don't notice. (Frey's syndrome is a neurological disorder linked to damage to the parotid gland and/or the auriculotemporal nerve in the face. It was an unexpected side effect of treatment for me.)

Challenges and suggestions for overcoming them

IN HOSPITAL

Learning to live with a real and constant fear

Take things one step at a time, and break those steps into smaller, manageable blocks. For example, CT Scan? I can do that. I can go down to the X-ray department; I've been there before. I can fasten my dressing gown, gather my stuff, walk out of the ward. Pay attention to everything. Wave at people I know. Take the stairs; that's easy, it's only stairs. They'll give me an injection; easy, they put needles in me all the time. Lie down on the table? I can do that. Breathe. And so on. It doesn't happen all at once. There's just this one thing that's happening right now, and I'm already inside it, so yes I can do it; I can stay in it; here I am.

Yes, I might die but I don't think it'll be today, it's not now, this is now and that's all that matters.

Being super-aware of each moment as it passed helped me. Being aware of my breathing. This may sound crazy to you if you've never meditated or done yoga or mindfulness training, but it is the simplest and most powerful thing in the world.

People will tell you that you have to be strong. Actually, you don't. There's no law that says you have to be anything. All you have to do is breathe. Sometimes it might be all you're able to do, but it's enough.

Coping with life in the goldfish bowl of a hospital ward

Get to know the people around you, both staff and patients. They are your friends and allies now. You won't have to look far to see people who are even worse off than you are, and that's a great antidote to self-pity. If you're well enough to move around, get out of the ward and go exploring. You need a change of scene.

Read, if you can. And I could do other things in short bursts: crossword puzzles and sudoku, which I learned how to do while in hospital. They helped a lot.

My notebook was the most helpful thing for me. I wrote everything down, whether it was practical or personal. When you're in hospital with a disease that needs professional input from a multidisciplinary team, as mouth cancer does, a bewildering procession of strangers will appear at your bedside, introduce themselves, pass on weird information, and wander off again. A lot of this will involve words you've never heard before and might not understand. Ask them to spell these words to be sure you've got them right. Write it all down, so that you can go over it later. Give it time to sink in. Record who they are, what their role is, what they tell you.

If you can't sleep and your mind is riding you like a demon, full of accusation, terror and regret, a notebook is a safe place to have a chat with yourself, or even a full-on shouting match. There may be things you can't say to people you love (or hate) but need to get out of your system. A notebook won't take offence or be frightened or break your confidence. It won't ever laugh at you or think less of you, no matter what you tell it. Actually, no one else will either, but it can feel safer to try these things out on a piece of paper first. And in the middle of the night there may be no one else to talk to.

Earplugs are a great help in hospital, as are music and books. The medical institution might control the externals, and your time, but *you* are still there, living your own fabulous inner life, undisturbed.

Hospital food is a definite challenge. It's shocking. So ask people who offer to help to bring in food that's fresh and healthy – things you like. Be specific about what you like and what you can eat. Do this when you're at home as well.

Ask the nurses to say you're not allowed visitors, when you don't feel like seeing people. Put a time limit on how long people stay. Don't wear yourself out being polite.

The mobile phone is a great tool in hospital. Get and send information by text, and turn the phone off when you don't want to communicate with anyone.

AT HOME AND BEYOND

Living with pain

Experiment with solutions. Bizarre things help me with pain. Strong-tasting juices like citrus or apple can displace pain in a peculiar way. Sweet things work for me too, but you have to balance that against the harm sugar does to your teeth and to your system generally; sugar is like poison for some people. If you have Frey's syndrome, like me, sweet things make your cheek sweat furiously, so have plenty of tissues to hand when you eat. Sweat will gather on your cheekbone and drip from your chin like a running tap. Really. It's bizarre.

Something cold held against the skin can help the pain. In more normal times, I'd put ice on a sore muscle or ankle, almost instinctively. Maybe it's a sign of how crazy my new internal wiring is, but it never occurred to me that it would work with the pain in my face and tongue – as though the new arrangement of my face is not part of me, even while the pain is driving me wild. It took a neurologist to suggest it to me, and it does help. Because of the size and shape of my scar, the bowl of a dessertspoon is about the right size and shape. I usually carry one around in my bag. If you hold it against the worst trouble spot, the cold can draw the pain away like a lightning rod.

I went through years of trying different types of medication, each exacting its own price. Some affected memory and concentration, and others played havoc with my digestive system. In the end I asked if it might be the case that I just had to learn to live with the pain and a doctor had the guts to say yes. After that I realised I had to get on with it.

There are some complementary therapies that help, like acupuncture or craniosacral massage. I found mindfulness training very helpful.

Exhaustion

People tell you that you'll be tired. They'll warn you about fatigue. You might still be shocked by how depleted, drained and empty you feel. Be patient with yourself if this happens. Give it time, get the best nutrition you can, and take it one step at a time. When you're absolutely wiped out, it's hard to imagine ever feeling better, or even what better might feel like. But time can be a magician.

There were times when I felt so low I could do nothing. There were times when I knew I should go out, or do some small thing for myself, but my sulky, despairing, self-pitying self would lie across the door and do its best to stop me. *You're too tired*, it would bleat. *Too weak. It's all too much.*

The trick was knowing when to listen and when to move that self out of the way and do the thing, whatever it was. Go upstairs. Flush the PEG tube. Paint my toenails. What amazed me was how much better I felt after battling to do the smallest thing, because every little thing was a tiny step towards recovery. And the small things paid off, in the end.

Adapting to disfigurement and physical limitations

A few days after the operation, my left leg was a pulpy purple mess. I had suspended all emotion on the subject for the time being. Then our five-year-old grandson came in to the ward when the dressing was being changed. His eyes nearly swallowed his face when he saw the leg. 'Did a shark bite you?' We all laughed, and that was that sorted. That scar was renamed the shark bite, and why not, when it was just as much a mark of survival as an actual bite would be?

In the days leading up to the operation, people were at pains to warn me about possible changes to my face. I couldn't imagine what it would be like, to have half a face. In the end I got tired of hearing about what *might* happen; I wanted to get on with it and deal with the reality of what would actually happen.

The reality was both better and worse. What mattered was function, not form. Day by day there were small improvements. I paid more attention to these improvements and to what I could do to make them happen than I did to how I looked or how people reacted. In fact, people notice less than you think they do. They have problems of their own.

My initial instinct was to hide, but what a waste of a second chance that would be. The next best thing would be to be as self-effacing as possible, right? So as no one will notice you? Well, no, actually, because then you're thinking about it all the time. I grew my hair. I wear brightly coloured scarves, big jewellery. Distraction works just as well, if not better, than hiding, and these things put me in a better mood.

Dry mouth

The only things that worked for me were water and Vaseline (after radiotherapy finished)[4]. I carried a bottle of water everywhere. It's easy to do and cheap. I

---

4. It is not recommended to use petroleum products while undergoing radiation treatment.

refilled old bottles from the tap. I have more saliva now; it's nearly back to normal but I still get random attacks of dry mouth, especially at night.

Difficulty eating

So much of our social life involves food: meeting people, family celebrations, parties etc. Sharing a meal is a basic part of our way of being with other people in the world. When this becomes problematic, it can be difficult.

I can taste and swallow, but I have restricted mouth opening and movement, fewer teeth and a sometimes dry mouth can get tricky. Those 'bite sized' tasties at parties are pretty much out of the question. Things that are too dry or hard are out of the question too. Give me a plate, a knife and fork and a lot of paper towels and I can tackle just about anything else. With sauce or soup there can be spillage, and not having sensation on my cheek or chin and part of my chest means that I can be wearing my dinner and not realise it. I say this to people upfront: I'm the original messy eater and if I have food on my face you have to tell me, because I won't know. Once it's been said it's not an issue.

Transport

Because I was in plaster and on crutches, I had to be driven to and from appointments all over town. We drew up a rota of friends and family and put it on a big wall chart in the kitchen. Some hospitals offer transport services, and the Irish Cancer Society now has two different supports for transport issues: Care to Drive and Travel2Care (see Resources and Contacts).

Coordination of appointments etc.

I got help with this from a person who was a huge support to me, a head and neck support nurse in St James's Hospital. She did all she could and went far beyond the norm, trying to set up appointments at times that actually made sense among all the other appointments in different hospitals, and in the matter of chasing down lost files. (When you have a lot of appointments with a lot of different specialists, even in the same building, files get lost.)

I think it would be of enormous benefit to mouth, head and neck cancer patients in general if everyone was assigned a case coordinator across all the diciplines and all the hospitals, from the time they're diagnosed until treatment is finished, and maybe a little beyond. If there's no one to do this for you on your team, someone in your family might take it on, although they won't have the same access to medical personnel or files. The summer of my treatment, one of my daughters, who was a student at the time, decided not to get a job but to look after me instead. It was a godsend. She handled everything, like collecting prescriptions, coordinating medications, doses, feeds, cleaning the PEG tube, all the various dressings, appointment cards and timetables. She drove me when other people couldn't, fielded phone calls and gave out information when we had it.

The cycle of different clinics and hospitals can be overwhelming at times. We made up a big chart listing every appointment, every treatment session, and who would drive to and/or from. It was good to be able to cross off each day when it was over, and to know we were one day closer to being finished.

Having to live by schedules imposed by institutions and clinics is a drain on your time and energy, and when you're this ill, time is all that matters and energy is in short supply. Bring a book with you, or a friend. Resign yourself to long periods of waiting. Leave the rest of the day free so that you're not under pressure and so that you can rest when you get home again. Make sure you bring more medications and/or food and water than you think you'll need, just in case.

Waiting for surgery was hard. Waiting for radiotherapy was harder. There was a long pause while they waited for various issues to resolve. Some medical people told me to be persistent and follow it up. Were they serious? Did they not know how wiped out I was? Not to mention the fear of antagonising people before they've even met you. Getting to St Luke's was a relief. It's hard to explain the positive impact of its atmosphere. I didn't have to explain myself; no one gave me a second glance. It was a safe place to practise going out in public. Having regular treatments there over seven weeks gave me a sense that we were all in it together, with the same goal in mind. I had physiotherapy there for my leg and it was brilliant.

Bring something of yourself with you to be your charm against what stalks you. Writing saved me: I brought it into the arena with me. A friend of mine, who has similar scars, made a point of always being dressed to the nines. No matter how ill she felt, she was without fail the most elegant person in the building. That was her way of saying, *Hey, this is me; I'm still here.*

When treatment finishes

Strange as it sounds, it can be hard to adapt to life when you're told 'That's it now.' These people have become like family; they've been your keepers. How will you manage without them? They've doled out your medication in strictly controlled circumstances; will you ever get the hang of it yourself?

Again, don't panic. It happens in stages: first when you're discharged from hospital, then when treatment finishes. Adapting to life outside the treatment regimen can be hard. It might help to know that most people, if not everyone, wobble a little at this stage. Be patient with yourself. If all the rigours of treatment don't bear down on you at once, getting better doesn't happen all at once, either.

Mouth care

- ➤ Carry water with you
- ➤ Use water as a mouthwash (avoid products with alcohol in them)
- ➤ Use a TePe brush for interdental cleaning

Neck and shoulder stiffness

Swimming really helps, and it builds general strength too. Consult your team before swimming.

Walking and being outdoors

Being out and about is good for the head, while actual walking will help rebuild your strength. Get used to taking your new self out in public.

Food and eating

EGG FLIP

My mother used to make us a ghastly concoction called an egg flip, which is basically a raw egg combined with milk and other stuff. It used to make us gag. There is a palatable version, though, which combines half a cup of milk and half a cup of orange juice with an egg, all whizzed up together. She used to add brewer's yeast, from the Irish Yeast Co. on College Street in Dublin. Amazingly, it's still in business.

NB: Do not use raw eggs if you are undergoing chemotherapy, are immune suppressed or at increased risk of infection.

Ingredients

1 egg

½ cup milk

½ cup orange juice

1 tsp brewer's yeast (if your stomach is up to it)

Method

Add the ingredients to an electric blender and blend on high for one minute. Alternatively use a hand blender and suitable jug.

LIQUADO

In Texas we used to sometimes kick-start a hot day with this tasty smoothie, which consists of lots of ice, orange juice and a banana, with or without an egg.

NB: Do not use raw eggs if you are undergoing chemotherapy, are immune suppressed or at increased risk of infection.

Ingredients

1 cup orange juice

1 banana

Lots of ice

1 egg (optional)

Method

Add the ingredients to an electric blender and blend on high for one minute. Alternatively use a hand blender and suitable jug.

Tip: If you are having ready-to-eat soup, try adding an egg. It is a simple way to boost nutritional value. When you're heating the soup in a saucepan, simply break an egg into the pan and stir together with the soup.

COLCANNON

Need I remind anyone about colcannon? Potato mashed with lots of milk or butter and pepper and salt; with handfuls of kale or cabbage chopped, cooked and thrown in, blended or not. Mash can be fortified with anything: yoghurt, cream, other root vegetables like parsnip, even fried onions, just to make it more interesting if you can't eat a whole lot else.

DIPS AND SPREADS

Dips like guacamole, hummus, pesto, tapenade etc. give maximum nutrition for minimum effort. It's good to have a few of these on standby to eat when you're hungry or if guests turn up unexpectedly. Eat with bread, crackers, carrot sticks, celery, strips of pepper etc.

STEWED FRUIT

Any fruit, alone or in combination with others, can be cooked until it's soft and mashable. Just peel and core the fruit if necessary, or use it whole if not. Put it in a pan with a little water and/or apple, orange, lemon or lime juice, depending on what you prefer and what you have in the house. Bring to a boil and simmer until soft. You can mash the fruit with a fork or use the hand blender to make a purée that's easy to swallow. If it's too tart, have it with yoghurt or sweeten it with honey or maple syrup. Greek style natural yoghurt has a lovely creamy consistency and will cool your tongue and temper the sharpness of the fruit.

Other things that helped

After I got home we discovered the joys of boxed sets and took up programmes like *The Sopranos*, *The West Wing* and *The Wire* (lent to us by friends) with enthusiasm. Now there's TV on the internet and Netflix, which do the same thing but don't cost as much.

One of the most helpful things anyone did for me came halfway through my treatment. A ward sister put me in touch with someone who had a different kind of cancer but had undergone similar surgery and treatment. It helped enormously to meet her and talk to her, and just to know I wasn't the only person on the planet this had happened to, because sometimes it feels like that. I was incredibly lucky in that we hit it off and became friends straight away. We could talk to each other in a way that you just can't with someone who hasn't been through it.

The Irish Cancer Society has a peer support programme. They can put you in touch with someone you can talk to. You might want to volunteer yourself, once you're through the treatment mill. Even if you don't want either of those things, it can be incredibly helpful to go to a cancer support centre (see Resources and Contacts) and meet other people, people with other cancers. I didn't think it would help me. I didn't see why it would, but it did.

Getting involved

I'm not a person who believes that everything happens for a reason. But if we can't always choose what life throws at us, we can choose how to respond. Getting involved in setting up a mouth cancer awareness campaign was important to me. I couldn't believe how prevalent the disease was, how devastating it could be and how little I or any of my friends knew about it (i.e. nothing). I couldn't believe how much easier it would have been to treat – for me and for the health service – if there had been more information out there and I had been diagnosed sooner.

As well as health promotion there are many different ways to volunteer with the Irish Cancer Society or other cancer support organisations and centres. When treatment finishes and you are free to get on with your own life again, you might prefer to walk away and not look back. There's absolutely nothing wrong with that. Do whatever's right for you, and enjoy it. But cancer is no friend of mine. I'll do whatever I can to stop it in its ugly tracks.

————◦————

PART THREE

FOOD, EATING AND RECIPES

Introduction

While you're in treatment, drugs can play havoc with your system. Your ability to open your mouth, chew and swallow, your sense of taste and your appetite might vary as you progress through treatment and your mouth reacts to surgery, radiation and/or drugs. A lot of us get trapped in a vicious cycle of constipation and diarrhoea. Everyone has to find the foods that help them, and those that don't.

Many mouth, head and neck cancer patients are encouraged to add full-fat food to their diet, because we tend to lose weight during treatment. A lot of these recipes pre-suppose that you've been given this advice. If you haven't, or if you have a medical reason for avoiding fatty foods, you can switch to low-fat options easily enough.

Diet and nutrition tips

- ➤ It is generally not a good idea to dramatically change your eating habits unless you are advised to do so by your medical team. For example you should not adopt an entirely vegetarian diet when you have been newly diagnosed with serious disease. The important thing is to get adequate nutrition to support your recovery

- ➤ Do not eat raw eggs if you are undergoing chemotherapy, as you may be immune suppressed and at increased risk of infection

- ➤ Nuts and seeds can be particularly difficult to swallow safely. You should get advice before including them in your diet

- ➤ Use honey sparingly as very frequent use will cause dental decay. Use it on porridge or on your fruit when eating a meal, but not in between meals. The same advice goes for sugar

- ➤ The single best kitchen tool is the hand blender. If you were to buy just one device, this one works hard, is easy to use and easy to clean. You can use a hand blender for smoothies and for soup, both of which will be vital elements of your diet. There's no real need for fancy recipes – just put your ingredients in a container such as a measuring jug and whizz them to the consistency you want.

➤ A juicer is necessary for harder fruits and vegetables like apples and carrots. Most juicers take longer to clean than it takes to drink the juice and when you're not feeling great it can all seem like too much effort. But it is worth considering this in the long-term.

———•———

RECIPES

Breakfast

HIGH-PROTEIN MILK (SJH)[5]
This can be used as you would normally use milk, in drinks, on cereals, in sauces and puddings.

Ingredients

570 mls full-fat milk

4 tbsp of milk powder (e.g. Marvel or Milk Made. You can find milk powder in most supermarkets)

Method

In a large jug add a small amount of the milk to the milk powder and whisk until the powder has dissolved into the milk. Add in the rest of the milk.

HIGH-PROTEIN, HIGH-CALORIE PORRIDGE (SJH)
Serves 1

Ingredients

200 ml high-protein milk (see recipe above)

35 g oatmeal

2 tbsp jam or honey

25 ml cream (optional)

Method

---

5. Recipes marked SJH are based on suggestions made by St James's Hospital, Dublin.

Make your porridge as normal using the high-protein milk. Stir in the cream and jam or honey before serving.

Smoothies

BASIC SMOOTHIE

A smoothie is easy to make. The base is a few heaped tablespoons of natural yoghurt (preferably live) with a couple of handfuls of berries – you can choose from blueberries, strawberries, raspberries, blackberries etc – and other fruit, depending on what you have and what you like. A banana will sweeten and thicken the smoothie. If you want more sweetness, add honey or maple syrup.

Ingredients

1 cup full-fat natural yoghurt or ice cream

2 handfuls of berries (any kind)

1 banana (optional)

Honey to taste (optional)

You can add high-protein milk (see recipe above) if you want to give it an extra boost

Method

Add the ingredients to an electric blender and blend on high until the desired consistency is reached. Alternatively use a hand blender and suitable jug.

———•———

Soups

BASIC SOUP

This recipe works with just about any vegetable, meat or combination of the two.

Basic Ingredients

Some form of onion, e.g. 1 yellow or red onion, 2–3 leeks, a bunch of scallions

1 tbsp light oil or butter

Meat and/or veg of your choice (the quantity will determine the thickness of the soup, this is a matter of taste and your ability to swallow. See recipe for green soup below.

800 mls stock (Either home-made or crumble a stock cube into 800 mls of

boiling water, stir well and add to the pot)

Optional: To thicken, add a cubed potato to the simmering vegetables and cook until the potato is soft.

Method

In a large saucepan, sweat the onion in the oil or butter until soft (about 5 minutes). Over a medium heat add the other ingredients, apart from the stock, and cook for about 5 minutes more. Add the stock, cover and simmer for around 30 to 40 minutes. Use a hand blender to blend to the desired consistency.

NB: Don't use a hand blender in a non-stick saucepan; it will destroy the non-stick coating. I learned this the hard way.

GREEN SOUP

This soup is surprisingly tasty, but subtle too. Keep it in a container in your fridge and heat it up when you want it. It is a great natural laxative, besides being full of goodies.

For the base, I use some or all of the following:

Ingredients

1–2 medium onions and/or 3–4 leeks and/or a bunch of scallions. Whatever you prefer.

1 tbsp light olive oil, sunflower oil or butter

A few stalks of celery and their leaves (use the whole bunch if you like)

2–3 green peppers, deseeded and chopped

1 head of cabbage, chopped

Black pepper

Parsley or other herbs

Method

Chop the onions and sweat them in the oil/butter in a large saucepan for about 5 minutes. Add a lot of black pepper and a handful of chopped parsley or other herbs if you have them.

Add the vegetables. Stir the lot together and add about 750 mls of stock. Simmer until the cabbage is cooked through, then whizz.

SPICY BUTTERNUT SQUASH SOUP

If you want something a bit fiery, try a soup like spicy butternut squash.

Tip: peeling raw butternut squash can be a challenge and quite wasteful. It's easier to peel when cooked. All you have to do is scoop the flesh from the skin with a spoon.

Ingredients

1 tbsp light oil or butter

1 small chilli pepper, deseeded and finely chopped (preferably red but green will do)

NB: Wash your hands immediately after handling. Don't rub your eyes, or you'll know all about it!

Fresh ginger (to taste), peeled and chopped

Fresh garlic (to taste), finely chopped or crushed

1 onion, finely chopped

1 butternut squash (or 4–6 medium sweet potatoes) peeled, de-seeded and chopped into small chunks

Method

Warm the oil in a large saucepan. Add the chilli, garlic and ginger and sweat for about five minutes while you peel, de-seed and chop the squash (or sweet potato) into small chunks. Add the squash to the other ingredients and cook for about another 5 minutes. Add about 750 mls of chicken stock or vegetable stock and simmer for about 40 minutes until the chunks of squash are soft. Blend using a hand blender or electric blender.

Variation: Replace half the stock with coconut milk. Yum!

POTATO, LEEK AND CELERY SOUP (Barbara Bolton)

1 tbsp butter

1 large onion, chopped

3 potatoes, peeled and cut into chunks

3 sticks celery, chopped

2 large leeks, carefully washed and sliced

2 chicken stock cubes

2 pints boiling water

2 cloves garlic, chopped (optional)

Parsley

Salt and black pepper

Method

Heat the butter in a large pot. Add the garlic if using. Over a medium heat add the vegetables and potato and make sure everything is coated in the heated butter. Dissolve the stock cubes in 2 pints boiling water and add to the pot. Bring to a boil, then reduce the heat and simmer until the vegetables and potato are soft. Add the parsley, salt and pepper. Blend the soup and enjoy!

HIGH-CALORIE, HIGH-PROTEIN SOUP (serves 2) (SJH)

Ingredients

200 mls condensed soup (e.g. cream of vegetable soup)

200 mls high-protein milk

2 tbsp cream

Method

Add the soup and high-protein milk to a saucepan over a medium heat and stir well. Bring to the boil, stirring all the time. Allow to simmer for 5 minutes. Pour the soup into a bowl and stir in the cream.

Optional: Add some grated cheese or cream cheese.

———◆———

Vegetables

ROASTED BUTTERNUT SQUASH

Butternut squash is a bit of a miracle, all by itself. My favourite way to cook it is really simple and unbelievably tasty.

Ingredients

1 butternut squash (any size)

1 tbsp butter (optional)

Cinnamon (optional)

Method

Heat the oven to 180° C. Cut the butternut squash in half, lengthways, and scoop out the seeds. Wrap each half in tinfoil and place them on a baking tray. Roast for about an hour, until the flesh is soft. Remove the tinfoil, scoop out the flesh, which should be as soft as butter. Add a little actual butter, if you must, and a sprinkling of cinnamon. Mash the mixture.

You can skip the butter and cinnamon and just mash the flesh with a fork and eat it straight away, if you prefer.

———•———

Eggs and cheese

Eggs are easy to cook and full of protein. It's hard to beat the flavour of a simple fried egg with mashed potato. Or try adding bits of ham, smoked salmon or smoked mackerel to scrambled eggs for a tasty breakfast or lunch. A soft-boiled egg mixed up in a cup with small pieces of bread or cooked potato makes a great snack. The yolk runs into the bread or potato and is extraordinarily comforting, if not exactly the most sophisticated thing you'll ever eat.

CHEESE SAUCE

Ingredients

30 g butter

30 g flour

500 mls (approx) milk

90 g cheese, grated (cheddar works best)

Grated nutmeg (optional)

1-2 tbsps grated parmesan

Salt and pepper to taste

Method

Melt the butter in a saucepan over a low heat. Add pepper, salt and nutmeg, to taste. Add a little parmesan if you like. Add flour and stir to an even consistency. Add the milk slowly, stirring all the time to avoid lumps. Keep stirring. When the liquid begins to thicken and is nearly boiling, take it off the heat and stir in the grated cheddar until melted. Add more parmesan for extra flavour, if you like. Delicious with meat, fish and vegetables.

———•———

Fish

Fish is a great alternative to meat. Its consistency is easier to manage with a damaged mouth. Properly cooked it flakes off and practically melts in the mouth. Small fishbones, on the other hand, are harder to deal with if your tongue isn't quite as flexible as it used to be. So, relatively boneless fish is what you're looking for. Fillets are best.

OVEN-BAKED FISH

The simplest way to cook fish is to wrap your fillet of fish in tinfoil with a knob of butter, a squeeze of lemon juice, pepper and whatever herbs you have (dill is great with fish, but anything will do). Roast in a hot oven (180° to 200° C) for about 15 minutes. Take it out and it's ready to serve.

It's just as easy to grill or fry, but some people object to the smell.

———•———

HORSERADISH MAYONNAISE

A teaspoonful of horseradish added to a cupful of mayonnaise goes beautifully with seafood like smoked salmon or prawns. This is a good lubricant for people with dry mouth, if you can tolerate the horseradish.

SMOKED MACKEREL PÂTÉ

Ingredients

450 g smoked mackerel, skinned and boned

140 g cream cheese

Juice and zest of 1 lemon

1 tsp of horseradish sauce, for extra bite (optional)

Method

Be sure no skin or bones remain in the mackerel fillets. Put the ingredients in an electric blender and blend for one minute. Alternatively use a hand blender and a suitable container.

———•———

Pulses and pasta

LENTIL AND MUSHROOM AU GRATIN (Hannah O'Driscoll)

Ingredients

For the lentils

2 tbsps oil

1 onion, chopped

1 carrot, chopped

2 sticks celery, chopped

1 clove garlic, crushed

8 oz. red lentils

1 pint water

2 tbsp shoyu (naturally fermented soy sauce)

For the mushroom filling

1 tbsps unrefined olive oil

8 oz. mushrooms, sliced

2 cloves garlic, finely chopped

3 tbsps parsley, chopped

To finish, 3 oz. cheddar cheese, grated

Sea salt

Method

Prehead the oven to 190° C.

Lentils: Heat the oil in pan and add the onion, carrot and celery. Cook for 10 minutes. Add the remaining ingredients. Cover and simmer for 50 minutes to 1 hour, stirring occasionally until lentils are tender.

Mushroom filling: Heat the oil in a frying pan. And the mushrooms and cook for 2 minutes. Add the garlic, parsley and sea salt to taste.

To assemble the gratin: Evenly spread half the lentil mixture in a medium oiled tin or greased oven dish. Spread the mushroom mixture on top, then spread the remainder of lentil mixture over the mushrooms. Top with the cheese and bake in a preheated oven (190° C) for 20 to 25 minutes, until golden brown.

From Heaven's Kitchen Cookbook (Yoga Society Ireland)

Puddings and desserts

FRUIT FOOL

Ingredients

Powdered custard (Bird's Custard Powder or similar)

Whipping cream (or half whipped cream, half Greek yoghurt)

Stewed fruit (apple, rhubarb, blackcurrant etc.) or mashed fruit (strawberry, raspberry etc.)

Method

Make the custard according to the packet instructions and allow to cool.

Whip the cream and stir it into the cooled custard. Add the stewed or mashed fruit, chill in fridge and enjoy when cool.

MILK PUDDINGS (RICE, SEMOLINA OR TAPIOCA)

Ingredients

50 g of rice (grain or ground), semolina or tapioca (Rinse the rice under cold running water before using)

600 ml full-fat milk

Sugar

Sultanas (optional)

Nutmeg (optional)

Cinnamon (optional)

Method

In a medium saucepan, gently simmer the rice, semolina or tapioca in the milk. Add the sugar when the grains are nearly cooked (about 10 minutes). Add optional ingredients, if desired.

EGG CUSTARD

Ingredients

3 eggs

500 mls milk

Sugar to taste

Cinnamon to sprinkle on top

Method

In a medium saucepan, bring the milk almost to the boil and then allow to cool slightly. Add sugar to taste. Beat the eggs in a bowl and add to the cooled milk. Pour the egg and milk mixture into a baking dish and sprinkle cinnamon on top, if using. (You could also divide the mixture between a few ramekin dishes to make single portions.) Place the oven dish in a larger baking dish or pan and pour warm water into the larger dish until it reaches halfway up the side of the smaller dish. Bake in a medium oven for about 30 minutes, until browned slightly on top. Allow to cool, and enjoy.

HOT CHOCOLATE (serves 1) (SJH)

150 ml high-protein milk (see recipe above)

2 tbsps whipping or double cream

3 tsps drinking chocolate powder

Cadbury Flake (optional)

Add all the ingredients to a small saucepan and heat until simmering, stirring continuously. Pour into a mug and top with cream and crumbled Flake.

HIGH-CALORIE JELLY (SERVES 3 TO 4) (SJH)

Ingredients

1 standard packet of jelly (any flavour)

200 mls boiling water

300 mls high-protein milk (see recipe above)

Method

Dissolve the jelly in the boiling water. Allow to cool, then add the high-protein milk and stir well. Leave the jelly to set. Serve with cream or ice cream.

———◆———

Notes from Anne L'Hénoret, Holistic Nutritionist

As a qualified holistic nutritionist I had ideas about feeding myself well post-surgery and even after radiotherapy.

To gain weight (things to eat when you can't chew or swallow well)

➤ Add calories and protein to soups by adding cream, coconut milk, puréed chickpeas, lentils or any canned beans. This requires no effort, and they can be tasty additions to shop-bought soups when you are too tired to cook. You really need protein to heal the skin, muscles and nerves after surgery. It is important not to just rely on cream, which contains a lot of fat. For example, use coconut milk to enrich a Thai chicken soup, or add puréed chickpeas to carrot and coriander soup. Any combination that appeals!

➤ Make very rich smoothies by combining full-fat milk, bananas, peanut butter, chocolate, or any combination of these. Nut butters are rich in protein to encourage healing

➤ Oily fish (salmon, mackerel, tuna and herring) are great for skin and nerve healing and are very easy to eat. I used to be vegetarian but I started eating fish again after my surgery for these reasons. You can even eat them cold out of a tin, if there is no one to cook for you

➤ Scrambled eggs are also fantastic. They're not a lot of work and they contain lots of good protein. I often used the microwave to cook them

When it becomes possible to eat out again

➤ Order the things that are easiest to eat (for example, soup, fish, mash, ice cream etc.) and save the hard or stringy foods like crackers or spinach or salad to eat at home. I found that allowed me to have conversations while out (once I had re-learnt to speak that is!) and avoid choking in public, which can be very tiring and frustrating. And don't worry about what other people think: most of them won't notice and the people you are with will think you are very brave to eat out and will be proud of you

If you have to avoid sugar to protect your teeth

Sugar is massively addictive, so if you cut it out you won't miss it for long. What you might miss is the choice of snacks and desserts when you are out, and also a sense of participation, as cake is a part of many celebrations

➤ Anything made with full-fat milk or yoghurt tastes rich and sweet to someone who has detoxed from sugar, so a full-fat latte or a Greek yoghurt can become treats. I never liked milky coffee before but now I do. When I had a very dry mouth, at the start, I used to flavour my Greek yoghurt with pure cocoa powder or coconut shavings. I also bought sugar-free chocolate in various flavours in the healthfood stores; there are several brands available. Occasionally I would bake using Xylitol

➤ Once I was less dry and I relaxed a bit about the sugar and my teeth, I set some ground rules to avoid getting carried away. For me, that means:

  · *No biscuits at work, ever. But something sweet at the end of a meal isn't so bad*

  · *I make exceptions for occasions and celebrations when there is a good cake around*

  · *I try to have yoghurt or ice cream with fruit or cake, as the calcium helps protect the teeth. A hot drink helps wash away the sugar quickly afterwards*

  · *I avoid crunchy or chewy sweets that really stick to the teeth*

I take things like savoury crackers, sugar-free chocolate, yoghurt, etc. with me when I'm travelling, as most corner shops, train stations, airports and the like mainly offer sweet snacks.

Finally, if you lose your sense of taste during radiotherapy, focus on the smell of the food, as you can still perceive that a lot of the time, and the textures. If it is really bad, remember you do need the fuel from food to recover. Don't give up on eating or eating well.

———— ◆ ————

PART FOUR

RESOURCES AND CONTACTS

Books

50 Essential Things To Do When the Doctor Says It's Cancer by Greg Anderson

What You Really Need to Know About Cancer by Robert Buckman

C: Because Cowards Get Cancer Too by John Diamond

Snake Oil and Other Preoccupations by John Diamond

Cancer Made Me a Shallower Person: A Memoir in Comics by Miriam Engelberg

Succeed by Heidi Grant Halvorson

Passionate Presence by Catherine Ingram

In Your Face by Lia Mills

The Emperor of All Maladies by Siddhartha Mukherjee

Take Off Your Party Dress: When Life's Too Busy for Breast Cancer by Dina Rabinovitch

The Tibetan Book of Living and Dying by Sogyal Rinpoche

First, You Cry by Betty Rollin

Moments of Stillness Sister Stanislaus Kennedy

The Power of Now: A Guide to Spiritual Enlightenment by Eckhart Tolle

A New Earth: Awakening to Your Life's Purpose by Eckhart Tolle

One in Three by Adam Wishart

Heaven's Kitchen Cookbook by Yoga Society Ireland

———— • ————

Booklets

Important Information About Radiotherapy to the Head and Neck by Denise MacCarthy, Dublin Dental University Hospital

Irish Cancer Society information booklets, available from the Irish Cancer Society or from cancer support centres:

- ➤ Understanding Cancer of the Head, Neck and Mouth
- ➤ Understanding Radiotherapy
- ➤ Understanding Chemotherapy
- ➤ Understanding Financial Advice

CDs and DVDs

The Irish Cancer Society produces DVDs on chemotherapy and radiotherapy. Contact them for more details.

- ➤ *A New Earth: Awakening to Your Life's Purpose* by Eckhart Tolle
- ➤ *Learned Optimism: How to Change Your Mind and Your Life* by Martin E. P. Seligman

Online resources

A note of caution regarding internet research: statistics don't mean a thing when it comes to individual cases. Remember that you don't always understand what's behind the figures you find on the internet. They may not apply to your case. Patient forums can be helpful, but remember that you don't know who you're talking to. No two cases are the same, and everyone's experience of cancer is different.

Irish Cancer Society: www.cancer.ie

The Irish Cancer Society is a charity that funds research and provides information about cancer, as well as offering many support services, such as the Care to Drive and Travel2Care programmes that help with transport or provide grants to help with the cost of transport. They also offer a peer support programme and operate the National Cancer Helpline (Freephone 1800 200 700), as well as publishing information booklets, running a buddy system, holding information days and much more. They can be contacted by e-mail or by phone (see listing below).

Irish Yoga Association: www.iya.ie

Macmillan Cancer Support (UK): www.macmillan.org.uk

Mood Gym: www.moodgym.anu.edu.au

Mouth Cancer Awareness Day (Ireland): www.mouthcancerawareness.ie

Mouth Cancer Foundation: www.mouthcancerfoundation.org

Ted Talks: www.ted.com/talks

Most TED Talks are inspirational. One that is particularly strong, on the concept of post-traumatic growth, is The Game That Can Give You Ten Extra Years of Life by Jane McGonigal.

Yoga Ireland: www.yoga-ireland.com

———•———

Organisations

Compiled by Róisín Whelan
(With thanks to the Irish Cancer Society for information supplied)

Ask your hospital or your GP where your nearest cancer support centre is and find out what they offer. Their services are usually free, and even though you might not think you need them or you feel awkward about going, they can really help.

CANCER RESEARCH IRELAND
Website: www.cancer.ie/research/why.php

CITIZENS INFORMATION
260 drop-in locations nationwide
Tel: 1890 777121
Website: www.citizensinformation.ie

EMPLOYMENT RIGHTS INFORMATION UNIT
Tel: 1890 201 615

HEALTH PROMOTION HSE
Website: www.healthpromotion.ie

IRISH CANCER SOCIETY
43/45 Northumberland Road, Dublin 4
Tel: 01 2310500, E-mail: helpline@irishcancer.ie
Website: www.cancer.ie

IRISH CLINICAL ONCOLOGY RESEARCH GROUP
Website: www.icorg.ie

IRISH HOSPICE FOUNDATION
Website: www.hospice-foundation.ie
Tel: 01 6793188

IRISH NUTRITION AND DIETETIC INSTITUTE
Ashgrove House, Kill Avenue, Dun Laoghaire, County Dublin
Tel: 01 2804839
Website: www.indi.ie

MACMILLAN CANCER SUPPORT (UK)
Tel: 00 44 207 8407840
Website: www.macmillan.org.uk

MEMORIAL SLOAN-KETTERING CANCER CENTRE (US)
Website: www.mskcc.org

NATIONAL CANCER INSTITUTE (US)
Website: http://www.cancer.gov/

WORLD CANCER RESEARCH FUND (UK)
Tel: 00 44 207 3434200
Website: www.wcrf.org

Cancer support centres

Leinster

ARC CANCER SUPPORT CENTRE
Arc House, 65 Eccles Street, Dublin 7
Tel: 01 8307333, E-mail: info@arccancersupport.ie
Website: www.arccancersupport.ie

ARC CANCER SUPPORT CENTRE
Arc House, 559 South Circular Road, Dublin 8
Tel: 01 7078880, E-mail: info@arccancersupport.ie
Website: www.arccancersupport.ie

ARKLOW CANCER SUPPORT GROUP
25 Kingshill, Arklow, County Wicklow
Tel: 0402 23590, E-mail: info@arklowcancersupport.com
Website: www.arklowcancersupport.com

BALBRIGGAN CANCER SUPPORT GROUP
74 Castleland, Parkview, Balbriggan
County Dublin
Tel: 01 8410116

BRAY CANCER SUPPORT & INFORMATION CENTRE
36B Main Street, Bray, County Wicklow
Tel: 01 2866966, E-mail: info@braycancersupport.ie
Website: www.braycancersupport.ie

CANTEEN IRELAND (young people's cancer support group)
Carmichael Centre, North Brunswick Street, Dublin 7
Tel: 01 8722012, E-mail: info@canteen.ie
Website: www.canteen.ie

CUISLE CENTRE
Cancer Support Group, Block Road, Portlaoise, County Laois
Tel: 057 8681492
Website: www.cuislecentre.com

DÓCHAS OFFALY CANCER SUPPORT
Teach Dóchas, Offaly Street, Tullamore, County Offaly
Tel: 057 9328268
Website: www.dochasoffaly.ie

DUNDALK CANCER SUPPORT GROUP
Phillipstown, Hackballscross, Dundalk, County Louth
Tel: 086 1074257

ÉIST CANCER SUPPORT CENTRE
5 Mount Clare Court, Carlow
Tel: 059 913 9684

GARY KELLY SUPPORT CENTRE
George's Street, Drogheda, County Louth
Tel: 041 9805100, E-mail: info@gkcancersupport.com
Website: www.gksupport.com

GREYSTONES CANCER SUPPORT
La Touche Place, Greystones, County Wicklow
Tel: 01 2871601, E-mail: info@greystonescancersupport.com
Website: www.greystonescancersupport.com

HOPE CANCER SUPPORT & INFORMATION CENTRE
22 Upper Weafer Street, Enniscorthy, County Wexford
Tel: 053 9238555, E-mail: info@hopesupportcentre.ie
Website: www.hopesupportcentre.ie

LAKELANDS AREA RETREAT & CANCER CENTRE
Multyfarnham, Mullingar, County Westmeath
Tel: 1850 719719, E-mail: info@larcc.ie
Website: www.larcc.ie

LITTLE WAY CANCER SUPPORT CENTRE
4 Woods Way, College Road, County Clane, County Kildare
Tel: 045 902996, E-mail: clane@littleway.org
Website: www.little-way.org

LITTLE WAY CANCER SUPPORT CENTRE
8 Stanhope Street, Athy, County Kildare
Tel: 059 8633725

TALLAGHT CANCER SUPPORT GROUP
Trustus House, 1-2 Main Street (opposite the Priory), Tallaght, Dublin 24
Tel: 086 4002736

WICKLOW CANCER SUPPORT CENTRE
1 Morton's Lane, Wicklow
Tel: 0404 32696

Munster

CARE CANCER SUPPORT CENTRE
14 Wellington Street, Clonmel, County Tipperary
Tel: 052 6182667
Website: www.cancercare.ie

CORK ARC CANCER SUPPORT HOUSE
Cliffdale, 5 O'Donovan Rossa Road, Cork
Tel: 021 4276688
Website: www.corkcancersupport.ie

KERRY CANCER SUPPORT GROUP
124 Tralee Town House Apartments, Main Street, Tralee, County Kerry
Tel: 066 7195560
Website: www.kerrycancersupport.com

LISTOWEL CANCER SUPPORT GROUP
Bedford, Listowel, County Kerry
Tel: 068 21741
Mid-Western Cancer Centre Mid-Western Regional Hospital, Dooradoyle
Limerick
Tel: 061 485163
Website: www.midwesterncancercentre.ie

RECOVERY HAVEN
5 Haig's Terrace, Tralee, County Kerry
Tel: 066 719 2122, E-mail: recoveryhaven@gmail.com
Website: www.recoveryhavenkerry.com

SLÁINTE AN CHLÁIR (CLARE CANCER SUPPORT)
Kilnamona, Ennis, County Clare
Tel: 1850 211630, E-mail: admin@clarecancersupport.com
Website: www.clarecancersupport.com

SOLAS CENTRE
South Eastern Cancer Foundation, 7 Sealy Close, Earlscourt, Waterford
Tel: 051 876629
Website: www.secf.ie

SUIMHNEAS CANCER SUPPORT CENTRE
2 Clonaslee, Gortland Roe, Nenagh, County Tipperary
Tel: 067 37403

SUIR HAVEN CANCER SUPPORT GROUP
Clongour Road, Thurles, County Tipperary
Tel: 0504 21197

YOUGHAL CANCER SUPPORT GROUP
161 North Main Street, Youghal, County Cork
Tel: 024 92353

Connaught

ATHENRY CANCER CARE
Social Service Centre, New Line, Athenry, County Galway
Tel: 091 844319
Website: www.athenrycancercare.com

BALLINASLOE CANCER SUPPORT CENTRE
Main Street, Ballinasloe, County Galway
Tel: 0909 645574

CANCER CARE WEST
Inis Aoibhinn Residence, University College Hospital. Galway
Tel: 091 545000

Or

CANCER CARE WEST SUPPORT CENTRE
72 Seamus Quirke Road, Galway
Tel: 091 540 040, E-mail: info@cancercarewest.ie
Website: www.cancercarewest.ie

GORT CANCER SUPPORT CENTRE
The Hawthorn, Ennis Road, Gort, County Galway
Tel: 086 3124220
Website: www.gortcancersupport.ie

MAYO CANCER SUPPORT ASSOCIATION
Rock Rose House, 32 St Patrick's Avenue, Castlebar, County Mayo
Tel: 094 9038407, E-mail: info@mayocancer.ie
Website: www.mayocancer.ie

ROSCOMMON CANCER SUPPORT GROUP
Vita House Family Centre, Abbey Street, Roscommon
Tel: 0906 625898, E-mail: vitahouse@eircom.net

SLIGO CANCER SUPPORT CENTRE
44 Wine Street, Sligo
Tel: 071 9170399
Website: www.sligocancersupportcentre.ie

TUAM CANCER CARE CENTRE
Cricket Court, Dunmore Road, Tuam, County Galway
Tel: 093 28522, E-mail: support@tuamcancercare.ie
Website: www.tuamcancercare.ie

Ulster

COOTEHILL COMMUNITY CANCER SUPPORT
Drumhose, Kill, Cootehill, County Cavan
Tel: 087 6220000

ÉIST, EAST INISHOWEN CANCER SUPPORT GROUP
Serenity House, 2 Montgomery Terrace, Moville, County Donegal
Tel: 074 9382874

GARY KELLY SUPPORT CENTRE
Monaghan
Tel: 041 9805100

LIVING BEYOND CANCER
Oncology Day Services, Letterkenny General Hospital, Letterkenny, County Donegal
Tel: 074 9125888

———◆———

INDEX